SPREAD THE JOY

Gaby Roslin

SPREAD THE JOY

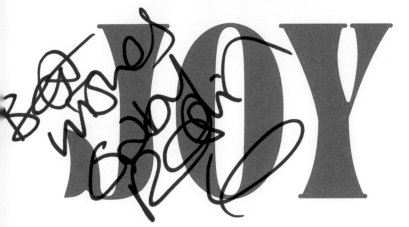

Simple, practical ways to make
your everyday life brighter

HQ
An imprint of
HarperCollins*Publishers* Ltd
1 London Bridge Street
London SE1 9GF

www.harpercollins.co.uk

HarperCollins*Publishers*
Macken House
39/40 Mayor Street Upper
Dublin 1
D01 C9W8
Ireland

10 9 8 7 6 5 4 3 2

First published in Great Britain by
HQ, an imprint of
HarperCollins*Publishers* Ltd 2023

Copyright © Gaby Roslin 2023

Gaby Roslin asserts the moral
right to be identified as the author
of this work. A catalogue record for
this book is available from the
British Library.

ISBN 978-0-00-855465-1

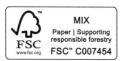

MIX
Paper | Supporting
responsible forestry
FSC
www.fsc.org   FSC™ C007454

This book contains FSC™ certified
paper and other controlled
sourced to ensure responsible
forest management.

For more information visit:
www.harpercollins.co.uk/green

Printed and bound in the UK
by Bell & Bain Ltd

Design & Art Direction:
Alice Kennedy-Owen

Publishing Director:
Louise McKeever

Managing Editor:
Clare Double

Editors:
Abigail Le Marquand-Brown and
Rachael Kilduff

Copy-editor:
Helena Caldon

Production Controller:
Halema Begum

Designers:
Lily Wilson and
Hannah Naughton

→ A note from Robbie Williams

What a great idea this book is. After all, apart from family and health I would put experiencing joy right up there with the most important treasures in my life. These days we are led by the nose down some pretty forbidding streets, pathed with anxiety, fear, self-loathing and a huge sense of 'what's-the-point?'. The point is joy; the point is love. It always has been. Outside of that it's all just 'things'.

We all know how to experience sadness – we're champions at it. For many, it's as easy and as natural as breathing. It seems like a terrible quirk of nature that to feel and experience happiness takes application, fortitude and a level of self-discipline, but so be it. As the old adage goes, you get out what you put in. I suggest opening these pages and putting in a little and seeing where it takes you. Bite size is the right size.

With this book Gaby has created something that should be part of the national education curriculum. After all, my need to understand the basics of the Industrial Revolution in fifth year pales into insignificance compared to the tools that this book provides. The three-field crop rotation has never, ever come up in any conversations I've had, and I doubt it ever will… Yet the desperate need to battle through mental illness and life's complex dark clouds is on everybody's tongues and minds.

Open yourself up to the possibility
that joy can exist for you.

Open yourself up to the possibility
that you just might deserve it.

Bless you, Gaby, for giving this wondering mind something loving and empathic to concentrate on. I always notice the nutrients friends and acquaintances give me: some are empty calories filled with starch, fat, salt and sugar, and then some are like Gaby Roslin – essential for your 5 a day.

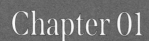
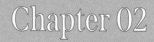

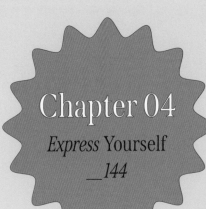
Contents

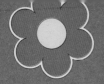

Introduction:
What Does Joy Mean to Me?

When I talk about joy, it makes me smile.

The definition of the word 'joy' is 'a feeling of great pleasure and happiness'; I have always believed that life can be full of joy, even at a very young age when I used to go to bed and change out of my pyjamas and into the next day's clothes because I couldn't wait for morning to come. My mum would come in every night and tell me I needed to sleep first and to get my pyjamas back on. I would say, 'But Mum, I can't sleep, and imagine what amazing things might happen tomorrow!' I used to stay awake in bed thinking and fantasising about all the magic that could happen; I would be there for hours imagining all sorts of things. Of course, the main thing I would think about was that one day my dreams would come true and I'd become a TV presenter.

From a very young age, people used to say that I was just like Pollyanna, after the unfailingly optimistic main character from Eleanor H. Porter's book of the same name. Pollyanna and I were very alike: she always played the 'Glad Game' – in which you find something to be happy about, no matter how bleak the situation is – and I did this too. If anything was making anyone sad, I would attempt to turn it into something that would make everyone happy. Pollyanna, of course, mainly used

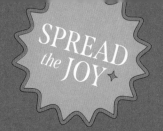

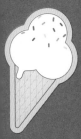

the Glad Game to boost her own spirits, but I didn't like the thought of anyone feeling sad. I wanted to try to fix them all, even as a very young child.

I was the most self-conscious, shy child and teenager you could ever meet. But I knew I always wanted to make people smile because they'd then feel joy. I realised that one of the most effective ways for me to do this was through my own laughter — I even learnt a way to make myself giggle because I knew it was contagious. I would lie down and kick my legs in the air and start laughing, then hold on to that feeling of uncontrollable giggles for as long as I could, so that I could pass it on to others. Other times, I would 'perform' for my family. Usually it was me 'presenting' a TV show, singing a song in a funny voice or doing an impression, but it would always end with me pretending to slip up or walk into something — that always did, and still does, make me roar with laughter. Through all of this, I learnt that if I helped people to smile and feel better, I would feel happier too. Over the years I have had many occasions where I haven't felt very joyful, but in those moments, looking for the joy in a situation has helped me enormously, as has making others feel happy, too.

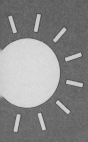

You might find it strange to hear how shy I was when
I was younger, knowing all of the things that I have
done in my career that many may consider to be a little
bonkers, but I was so shy that I would be loath to do
anything that someone would judge me for or think
I was 'different' for doing, unless I was performing.
Knowing that I wanted to make people smile meant it
didn't take me long to work out what I wanted to do
in the future. In fact, from the age of three I watched
a children's TV show called *Blue Peter* and I decided
that's what I wanted to do. So if anyone ever asked me
what I wanted to be when I grew up I would always
say the same thing: I want to be a TV presenter and
a performer. I loved and still love TV, films, theatre
and entertainment – TV has made and still makes me
happy. So in my mind it was obvious that this would be
the best way for me to make others happy too.

For years and years after I made it onto TV in 1987,
journalists used to ask me, 'Why are you always happy?'
Rather strangely, I used to apologise for being happy
and joyful. Then in 1997, when my mum died at a young
age, I made myself a promise that I would never again
apologise for being happy or joyful. I refused to say
sorry any more for feeling that life is precious, or
for trying to help others feel joy. Today, I laugh, skip,

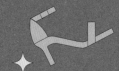

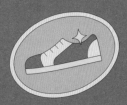

dance and sing without restraint and, whenever I can, I encourage others to do the same. We all have the power inside of us to feel and spread joy, and if we can do it, well, why not?

Joy is something that I feel is vital for helping us to cope with life. It's a tough old thing to try to grab hold of, especially when life can be very difficult, but it's much easier to do so when someone takes your hand and helps you. This book is that hand — which I'm extending to you now. The words within it have been written by me, for you, with love and joy, in the hope that you receive them in the same way. I'm confident that if you approach them with an open heart, the strategies within this book will help you to find joy, too.

In *Spread the Joy*, I want to introduce to you the five things that I consider most important in living a more joyful life — call them leaps towards feeling and spreading joy. The best thing about these 'leaps' is that none of them requires anything above and beyond from you — they are so powerful, yet you don't need any money or equipment to do them. They only require you to decide to do something that will help yourself and others; they might feel a little bit out of the ordinary, but that's a good thing!

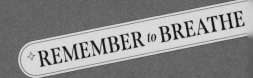

REMEMBER *to* BREATHE

For years those who have played by certain rules have been held as shining examples in our society, which is why we, in turn, have begun to feel secure when we follow them, when no one is looking at us – when we are being 'good'. This book will assist you to slightly step outside of your comfort zone. I will encourage you to act with as much carefree abandon as you probably did when you were a child – long before you learnt what it meant to feel scared of what others thought of you – which is something I try to do every day now. These things might make you feel a little daft to start off with, but stick at it! What I'm going to say to you now is what I wish I could have let my younger self know when she was feeling very shy and awkward and when she didn't want to do things that were out of the ordinary. And here it is... More often than not, no one will give a thought to what it is that you're doing, or even care. Instead, they're probably just worrying about what they're doing and what others might think of them.

Joy in life really comes from the times when we decide to step out of the ordinary – to make every day fun. And if having fun means that people start looking at you – well, who cares? People will be looking at you and hopefully smiling, so you'll be spreading the joy without even having to try. Trust me when I say that if you feel joy in your heart, there's nothing better than sharing it and spreading it, and knowing this will help you to throw off any self-consciousness.

I'm not trying to be preachy in these pages – I know some things will work for you while others won't, and that there is nothing within this book that you MUST do – but if there's even one thing in here that you can adopt in your life to make you feel better, wouldn't that be great?

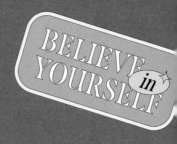

Today's Tiny Tasks

Now, please let me introduce you to your Tiny Tasks,
which you will find scattered throughout the chapters.
You may very well wonder what on earth these are, so
let me explain. These are just things that I would love
you to try; simple ways to get joy into your life. These
are only small but they can lead to bigger, fully grown
Tasks. I just want you to feel okay in trying these out, as
they won't hurt – please trust me on this. If you have a
pencil, this is the part where I give you full permission
to tick these off. Each and every time you complete a
Tiny Task, pop a tick next to it or even write the word
'Done' beside that task. When you look back, imagine
the thrill you'll have when you see all of those new
Tiny Tasks either completed or at least attempted.
Remember, no one is judging you. No one is giving
you one of 'those looks'. Just give it a go.

**I'll be with you all the way through the book,
so let's do this together.**

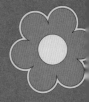

Chapter_

It Starts
Inside of_

01

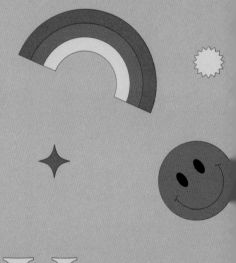

You

In order for **YOU** to be able to start spreading *joy* to **OTHERS**, we need to start with **YOU**.

We all spend so much time worrying about what other people think, but you know what, it really doesn't matter. What matters is what's going on inside of you. If you don't feel good in yourself it will be very hard for you to spread the joy to others. *How can you give something to someone without first feeling it yourself?*

So, how are you coming to this book? How do you feel right now?

Awkward?

Self-conscious?

Shy?

Embarrassed?

Okay?

Pretty crap?

Unhappy?

Or maybe not bad, but could be happier?

If you're able to, please take a moment to really become aware of how you feel inside.

No matter how good, bad or average you feel, you have the power inside you to make yourself feel better (or even better than you do now!). If you're already feeling good, write down how that feels physically in this moment. It might just be something as simple as your shoulders have dropped or your breath is calmer. Now think about what helped you to feel this way. It may be that someone smiled at you, or you ate your favourite breakfast this morning, or your partner was being supportive about some issue. Whatever it is, enjoy the moment and note down what it was that helped get you there. In this book, I'll frequently be asking you to draw on some of your favourite things, so noticing where these present themselves is a great start.

If you're starting this book feeling not so brilliant, *stick with me.* I *truly* believe you will find something in here that will help you. So, let's begin this 'finding joy' lark together. Your actions can help you to feel joy and pass it on to others. *Let's go!*

How *are* you?

How do we begin to feel joyful in ourselves?

In the first instance, I'd like you to start simply by asking yourself:

> How are you *feeling* today?

The reason I say this is because we all ask others how they are feeling, but we rarely check in with ourselves. When we are asked this question by others, we'll often instinctively say 'I'm fine', or 'Not too bad' (do we even realise when we're saying these phrases or even notice how they actually sound?), without even thinking about the question. When was the last time you thought about how you are really feeling when someone asked you that question? So, again, I'll ask,

> How are you?

... and I want you to tell me a truthful answer this time.

Don't judge yourself when you reply. If you're feeling absolutely dreadful because you've just had a raging argument with your children for the third time this week, say it! If you're feeling absolutely brilliant because your partner has just gone on holiday for a week and you're already envisaging how much excellent crappy TV you're going to get to watch on your own, say that! Don't judge yourself by your answer – no one else besides you will hear it.

● Be honest with yourself

Next, I want you to ask yourself how you're feeling every morning.

Tell yourself if you're feeling rubbish, or if you're feeling happier than you've felt in weeks. Checking in with your emotions will allow you to determine what it is that you need in order to make you feel joy today. Sometimes you'll already be feeling joyful, and in identifying that you can start to feel grateful for your happiness. Please never forget that fake joy is a definite no-no, because people can always tell when the joy you're displaying isn't real – most of all, you!

So, start by being truthful with yourself. In time, you can try searching for an honest answer when others ask you how you're feeling, too – you really never know what sort of candid conversation may then open up. Or indeed, when someone's kindness in response to YOUR sadness might be all that YOU need to make you feel joy again.

> *Joy comes from within, so the more you feel truly happy within yourself, the more you'll start to be able to radiate it outwards.*

• Listen to *your* body

I spoke to someone recently who told me that she feels as though she tries so hard to make everyone happy that she never leaves time for herself. I told her to stop and listen to her body, and ask it what it was that she really needed. After some time reflecting, she said she needed not to smile. I'm of the opinion that if something isn't making you feel happy, you should stop doing it, so I told her that it was fine to not smile, that she really didn't need to, or shouldn't feel that she needs to do so in order to make other people happy. A few days later, she put this into practice and a man who had seen her not smiling said to her in the street, 'Oh come on, love, it might never happen.' She stopped and told this man the truth, that she was taking a moment for herself not to smile, and he apologised.

When met with this comment (and might I just add here that passing judgement like this really is NOT OKAY, or the way for you to spread joy), many of us might feel the need to smile, or apologise, or just walk away in anger and be left feeling really frustrated about the encounter all day. But in being honest, she turned it around. She also said that when the man apologised, she couldn't help but smile – for herself this time.

I am certainly not saying that being honest to someone who insults you will always result in an apology that will leave you smiling – no way! But I am saying that listening to your body, being honest about what it needs, and informing other people of those needs, will leave you feeling lighter.

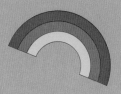

✳ Remember to breathe

One of the most important things you can do to make yourself feel more joy is breathe. I know what you're thinking: 'Gaby has lost the plot, I breathe constantly, otherwise I'd be dead!' This might sound like a whole bunch of crazy loony stuff, but honestly, taking the time to consciously breathe rather than just letting our body do it on autopilot is so valuable.

Let me be clear here, when I talk about taking a moment to breathe I'm not referring to the sort of breathing that you might expect to do in a yoga session. I don't want you to sit cross-legged and chant 'Omm' (although, goodness me, yoga can really help you feel more joy). I'm talking about simply consciously starting to think about your breathing. In our incredibly busy lives, we rarely find time to pause and do just that. Everyone has places to go and people they need to see. I know that I, for one, try to fit as many things as humanly possible into one day and would 'forget' to stop and breathe if I didn't remind myself. But we simply can't live like this and remain joyful – we need to have some time to ourselves. And that's where breathing comes in.

I know that I, for one, try to fit as many things as humanly possible into one day and would 'forget' to stop and

BREATHE

if I didn't remind myself. But we simply can't live like this and remain joyful - we need to have some time to ourselves.

1

Let's try this together.

2

Stop. Take a deep breath in. Breathe in as far as your lungs will let you.

3

Hold the breath for a second or two.

4

Now, let it all out slowly with an open-mouthed sigh.

It might feel like you've just done something that's beyond simple – maybe you even feel as though you've done nothing at all – but I promise you that the effects of breathing in this way can be revolutionary, especially if you do it whenever you're feeling a little overwhelmed.

Breathe in, and let out a huge sigh again.

Now, tell me, what was it that you were you thinking about when you were breathing?

I know that when I take in a deep breath, I often think about nothing more than how full my lungs are feeling, then how good it feels to have let out all that air.

In thinking about this, rather than about what needs to happen in my day, I'm disconnecting from my busy mind and living more in the moment.

In other words, by *breathing* you're taking a moment to just be here, with yourself.

Breathe and smile

Now, if you feel like you're ready to take the next step, just breathe in and out again, but this time when you breathe in, try a smile. You don't need to do a huge cheesy grin, I mean just a gentle smile. I'm going to talk a lot about smiling in this book for a very simple reason: when you smile you automatically feel happier. I truly believe that a smile is one of the most powerful weapons that you can wield when you want to feel more joy, so let's use it more. In fact, more and more studies have shown how powerful a smile can be (more about those studies later).

Start identifying moments in which you're feeling a little bit overwhelmed and perhaps not very joyful at all. In these moments, pause and use your two very simple tools: a smile and a breath.

→ *Spread the word*

Once you've mastered this, it's time to start identifying when others might need to breathe, and to get them to breathe and smile with you.

I have a friend who is always running herself into the ground trying to juggle children, work, a marriage breakup and looking after her elderly parents. When she's struggling, she always rings me to ask me to remind her to breathe. When she really can't cope, I suggest she sets a gentle smile on her face and then breathes in and out. She says that the simple act of me reminding her to do this helps her reset.

Sometimes we all need someone to give us 'permission' to take time out for ourselves. So when you next see a friend or family member who is doing too much, ask them to breathe with you. Tell them how important it is for them to take a moment for themselves. That is how you start spreading the joy.

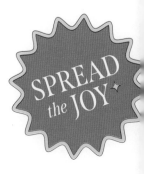

SPREAD
the JOY

• Believe in yourself

Believing in yourself is a key factor behind feeling joyful, but it's often assumed that in order to believe in yourself you need to have confidence – which is something many people struggle with. I am speaking to you as someone who has always been shy; as someone who has had, and at times still has, not a huge amount of confidence. Confidence is a skill you can learn – you don't have to be born with it – but it can be difficult to master. And if you can't, don't panic, just keep working on it – being shy, or having a lack of confidence, has never stopped me from following my dreams nor, by extension, has it stopped me from feeling joyful.

So how can I convince myself to do the thing when these feelings of doubt or shyness wash over me? I have been known to talk out loud to myself, and I have also been known to look in a mirror and tell myself that I can do it, that I've got this. If I really want to fire myself up, I'll sometimes even say to myself before walking out, '**Here I come!**' I am also incredibly lucky to be in a job I have always dreamed of doing and still love to do, but there have been tough times and my confidence has sometimes been chipped away by these.

Instead of thinking that someone else will be cleverer, more interesting, happier or better than me, I breathe and I smile. I wipe those unhelpful scenarios from my mind and tell myself that I AM capable, and that those people will likely be thinking the same thing that I am right now. And it always makes me feel better.

You can do this, too. The next time you're starting to think that you can't do something, pause, look in the mirror, and tell yourself that

YOU CAN.

If there's no mirror around just hold that feeling in your gut and your heart and mind. Before you start thinking about all of the things that could go wrong, breathe and instead think about all of the *wonderful* things that could and can go right. Focus only on the here and now. Know that you can do it. When you do the thing that you've been scared to do, and don't let your fear stop you, joy will wash over you in waves.

✻ Appearances matter

_____ *but not in the way that you think...*

So we've started by talking about working on yourself from the inside. We've spoken about breathing and being honest with yourself, and about using positive affirmations to believe in yourself, but getting joy from these things can often take practice. We're not always hit with a burst of positive emotion the first time we try.

So what happens if you're due to leave the house and head off somewhere, and you're not sure that you want to go because you're feeling rubbish about everything? Some people might think that what I'm about to say is silly, but hear me out.

I do believe that one of the things you can concentrate on when you're feeling this way is your outfit.

→ *Colour lifts you*

It's fascinating how we've all been pushed into a plain, safe, dark clothing corner because we've been told it makes us look 'elegant' and 'sophisticated' day or night, or we dress conventionally at work because 'that's what I always wear'.

I remember hosting *Motormouth* on Saturday mornings, which was for kids so we always wore crazy colours and fun outfits, but when I started on a nationwide breakfast show (*The Big Breakfast*), I thought I should look 'more grown up' and wear duller, more serious clothes. However, our editor (Sebastian) said it was important to lift people's moods at breakfast time, and that colour helps do that. He wasn't wrong.

Even a little injection of colour in a drab outfit can help lift your mood, which will, of course, help you feel more joyous, and there are scientific reasons behind this – the most important being the fact it hits 'release' on the hormone dopamine (known as the feel-good hormone) within our body. When one of my beautiful friends died aged only 40, she asked if we'd all wear bright colours to the service, especially pink. She wanted brightness and smiles, and choosing colour certainly lifted our moods a tiny bit. I smile whenever I think about her.

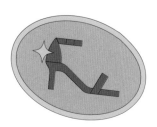

This feel-good hit that we get from colour is something that, if you are anything like me, you probably will have understood without realising it when you were younger. I imagine that we'll each have chosen wild and wacky colourful outfits that expressed how we felt as children, but then something crazy happened: we would be very concerned about what others might think of us. We saw what other people were wearing and thought that we probably shouldn't wear things that went against the grain anymore. We listened to that inner voice that doubts our choices, or that nasty person who says, 'Oh, that's not your colour, is it?'

Well, I now give you full permission to ignore them and your own insecurities. Yes, you're probably thinking, 'Ignoring my insecurities is hard!', and I know, and understand. But the best way for you to overcome these is for you to pick colours that you really, genuinely love, and to own your decision to wear them, and celebrate wearing them. Wearing an outfit confidently will allow you to feel much stronger, and for those nagging insecurities to get much quieter.

→ *Add a splash of colour*

If you don't want to go full colour, you can just add little splashes here and there. So here are some simple tips for how to do this.

Open your cupboards, and instead of looking at the types of clothing you have, look only at the colours that you have to wear. I bet the first colour you'll see is black – our wardrobes are full of it – so move past that. What's left? If it's white, push that to the side with the black. If it's beige, that doesn't count either. Once you've removed everything from your sight that's black or neutral, you will hopefully be left with some items of clothing that are truly colourful.

Choose one of these items, and only now can you take out an item that's black, white or beige to match with it. See how you've created a different look already? It really is that simple. Not only have you potentially got out of a negative outfit spiral, you've also pulled together an altogether more joyful ensemble.

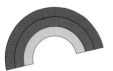

PICK COLOURS THAT YOU REALLY, GENUINELY LOVE, AND OWN YOUR DECISION TO WEAR THEM.

ANYONE
CAN
WEAR
PINK

→ *Then add more!*

But what if you don't have any colour in your wardrobe? Well, now is the time to introduce some. If you're not sure where to start, nearly all surveys on colour say that blue is everyone's favourite. We associate it with blue skies, oceans and lighter days.

Why not borrow a blue item from a friend and see how it feels?

Why not wear a blue top with your favourite pair of jeans?

Pink is also popular – it's the colour of love and romance, of passion… and also innocence! I love that it can be either naughty or nice. I do realise that not everyone will want to wear this colour, as some still believe it's 'only for females', but I reject this idea altogether. Please don't get me started on that debate…In my opinion,

anyone can wear pink.

And while we're talking about annoying rules, redheads can wear pink too – and red. All you need to do is choose a colour that you like, not what you think someone else would like. If you've always loved the colour orange, wear it. Sod the colour rules. In fact, forget the rules entirely! Rebel, wear what you want, and while you're at it, wear colour. It will lift your spirits.

I bet when you started reading this part of the book you thought that I would be taking you on a huge journey? No, it's always about keeping it simple. So pop on that colour, enjoy wearing it and relish that dopamine hit.

$\rightarrow$ *Don't overthink it*

NEVER think about what you're going to wear to meet your friends, to that wedding, or to work, etc., for too long in advance.

If you do, you'll start creating pictures in your mind of how you're going to look, and you may end up feeling miserable that you don't look like that, instead of just enjoying the moment.

Sometimes your outfit is the reason why you're feeling a bit rubbish – or rather, how you are feeling when you put it on. The moment I try on something that I have planned to wear and it just doesn't work can be the undoing of me. It doesn't matter if my husband says it looks great, if I'm in the mindset where I'm looking for things that are wrong, and I've decided that this outfit is everything that's wrong, there is no way I am going to wear it. This isn't just a woman thing; this is something that we all feel. And it really does sap your joy.

So reframe that mindset. Take a moment, stop, breathe in and out slowly and imagine how you want to feel. Be honest with yourself – if this is a 'I feel crap and lumpy' day then, please, don't grab a black outfit out of the wardrobe. Seriously. For years we have been told that black slims us down, and while technically this might be true, black can also bring down our moods.

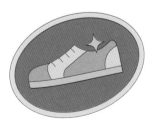

Commit to your choice

I have managed to make myself feel brilliant wearing outfits using this method, even those that are a bit 'out there'. I remember wearing an outfit that clashed ridiculously once, one that I really liked but felt self-conscious in, until I reminded myself that I loved how it looked. So I decided to label my outfit choice – I called it 'Patt Clash', and celebrated the experience of wearing it. Patt Clashes are now mainstays within my wardrobe – whenever I wear them, I shout, **'Patt Clash comin' a'tcha!'** at my family and friends. And because I am confident in the fact that I like what I've decided to wear, when anyone says that they're not sure of the colours or patterns that I've combined, I smile and tell them that it's a Patt Clash. It doesn't bother me. They're often flummoxed, but more often than not, they also smile when I say so. (In case you're wondering what 'Patt Clash' stands for, it's PATTern CLASH! And if I ever meet the tennis player Pat Cash, he may get slightly confused if I shout that at him.)

So, no matter what you have on (even if you don't think that it's your colour or your pattern), if you wear it confidently, I can guarantee that most people will do nothing but smile at you – even if it's the brightest of outfits. In fact, I have a neon outfit or two (I'm winking and smiling as I write that because I may have more than a couple) and each and every time I wear them someone says, 'Oh wow, that's colourful.' They may not like the colour themselves, but it makes them smile. In fact, so often, when I wear one of the very bright things from my wardrobe, someone will say, 'I wish I had the confidence to wear that colour.' Well, if you don't let your own self-doubt and belief that someone will say something awful get in your way, you bloody well can.

Today's Tiny Tasks

These Tasks are about colour. I would love to be there holding your hand and looking into that mirror with you right now as you're doing this – but not while you're getting dressed, as that would be too weird.

1

Wear one colourful item. It can be absolutely anything – from a top, some socks, a scarf or even a bag. Now walk around your home with it on and catch sight of yourself in various mirrors, and as you do, smile.

2

Wear that item outside of your home. You can just pop out if you don't yet feel confident, and you really don't have to go far unless you want to.

3

Wear one colourful piece of clothing to work, or to meet up with friends. I am sure they'll make the usual remark: 'Wow, you never wear a colour, you look great!' Get a selfie in your colourful outfit.

Once you do this, there's no going back to all black – unless you want to mix it up from day to day, of course, but even then, please pop a little splash of colour somewhere just for me.

IT'S A MYTH THAT PEOPLE ARE EITHER BORN SPORTY OR NOT SPORTY. I HAVE FOUND THE THINGS THAT I LOVE TO DO TO KEEP ME FIT, AND I DO THEM WHENEVER I CAN.

✹ Move as often as you can

When I was at school, I couldn't touch my toes, I couldn't play sports and I wasn't picked for the rounders team by anyone who was captain. I was never sporty at all. I could sprint, and that was it. It was such a struggle that it often made me feel even shyer than I already was. That awful moment when the sports teachers would say, 'Right, who wants to play rounders?' would make my body quiver, and I would want the ground to open up.

Over the years, though, I have learnt to hugely love fitness and the joy it brings me. And guess what? I can now touch my toes, I can hit a rounders ball and I love to work out every day of the week. It's a myth that people are either born sporty or not sporty. I have found the things that I love to do to keep me fit, and I do them whenever I can. I am nowhere near the best, nor do I pretend to be or want to be, but I can keep up with myself.

So there we go – I am proof that you can feel even fitter than you did when you were a child. Please don't let anyone tell you otherwise (least of all yourself. In fact, if you're telling yourself that now, go and give yourself a talking-to in the mirror).

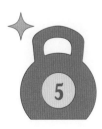

→ *Find a type of movement that makes you smile*

Now, I'm NOT going to tell you which exercises you should try to do. Oh no, this isn't that kind of book – and exercise is so subjective that you might not like what I do anyway. I bought my best friend some bands (the stretchy type intended for workouts, not Coldplay or Take That); she gave them a try once and told me that she never intended to do them again (they really did go down a treat). But she said using them made her rethink how she would like to keep fitter and keep moving. She now does Pilates, and says that each time she leaves a class she smiles. It's contagious, in a good way, and she believes it's changed her outlook on life. So even if you don't enjoy the exercise you start off with, you might find something that you like as you keep trying new things. Exercise fills me with joy, and it will fill you with joy too, if you find the right kind for you.

There are, of course, so many studies that prove how important and valuable exercise is. I know many people who tell me they just don't want to hear how vital it is in our lives, but let's keep to the basics. Exercising in the right way can and will make you feel better, stronger and healthier. People who exercise regularly also lower their risks of developing many long-term chronic conditions such as heart disease, strokes, type 2 diabetes and some cancers.

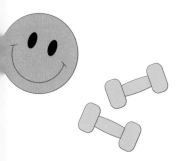

→ *Start slowly*

If you have never exercised before (apart from walking, jogging or swimming), it's a good idea to go for a quick medical check-up first, as I don't want you doing something you really shouldn't. If you know you're okay to give it a go, though, why not try exercising now, even if it's been years since you last did? Don't push yourself to do what you really can't. Don't try to keep up with your friend because they can do 30 press-ups and begin each day annoyingly Lycra-clad and sweatband-covered (wait, do people still do that? Oops… I think I just ventured back into the 80s for a moment). Just move.

Try just a short workout which involves some weight-bearing exercises – that's where your feet and legs support your weight, such as jumping, walking fast on the spot, playing tennis or dancing – which are really good for your bones. Once you're comfortable doing that, try exercising a little bit longer and a bit harder, but only when you're really ready. I like to combine weight-bearing exercises with resistance exercises that use weights – just dumbbells that I've had for years – because I know from personal experience that if I push myself a little bit more, it makes me feel so great!

Of course, sometimes I don't want to exercise. There are times when I really don't feel 'in the mood', but I promise – yes, a real promise – that once I do even a 15-minute workout I feel better. Your exercise doesn't have to be full on, and it definitely shouldn't be to begin with; just a few little gentle movements can make you feel better. And make sure that you start now; not tomorrow or Monday, now. Put this book down, get up and move your body.

Check out the amazingly helpful online tutorials that I have found over the past few years, such as those that I've listed in the Tiny Tasks on page 51.

It's very

annoying

when

someone

tells you

something,

isn't it?

But trust me,

exercise lifts your spirits,

and you will feel
joyous afterwards.

Today's

Tiny

Tasks

1 Stand up and stretch
your arms up above your head.
That's how I would love you to start;
imagine you're finishing off a huge yawn.
Grab two tins from your kitchen or two water
bottles and hold one in each hand. Keep your
elbows in to your side and curl the weights up
to your chest and then down – you can even
march whilst doing it. Oh yes, and sing a song
and, if you can, try to smile! You may feel
daft, but that's part of it. Curl up
10 times and then stop.

2

Squat as many times as you feel you can.
Build those squats by a couple more each day.

3

Watch a workout on YouTube. Yes,
this is me telling you to just watch one
first, BUT then do it along with the instructor.
Do it. I can highly recommend Caroline Girvan,
Alice Liveing and, of course, everyone's favourite,
the Body Coach himself – Joe Wicks. These are all
people who I have followed over the past few years, and
I love what they do. They really know their stuff.
Committing to doing one of these workouts regularly
will be a brilliant way to help regulate your mood – I
now try to do one five times a week, but even doing
one once or twice a week, or noticing when your
mood drops and trying to slot in some
exercise, will be hugely beneficial.

You don't need any fancy equipment to get going - just yourself.
Have a go at the above and see how much better you feel.

• Redefine success

I heard some great news about an old friend this week. They recently found out something truly amazing has happened to them and their business. They have spent years doing everything and anything they can to earn money while coming up with other business ideas, and always felt that they had that 'special idea' that would stick. And this week it finally happened.

Their news was so exciting that when I heard it I screamed with joy and love. But another friend, who had been there to hear the news, said they found it tough to hear about this person's success because they felt they hadn't had any themselves. They gave me a look that said, 'Don't tell me I have success because I am lucky to have what I have,' but I wasn't going to say that.

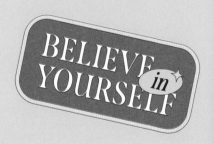

→ *What is success?*

People seem to want to be a success, but success isn't something that can be objectively defined. Is it:

Money?   Fame?

Having more flowers in your
garden than your neighbours?

                              Going on an expensive holiday?

I think we all spend too much time beating ourselves up thinking we haven't made a success of this or that when success doesn't really mean anything at all on its own. We define it.

Do you know what I believe? You might not be a Premiership footballer or a movie star, or at the top of the business that you've been in for years, but you are a success. Not because you have lots of money, or all the friends, or good grades, but because, quite simply, you are here. You're reading this right now. You're a living, breathing human being, and for that, you are successful.

We can all reach our potential, because we define what that potential is. One friend's massive success does not have to be the same as your success. And just because they've had that success, that doesn't mean your ideas have no validity in the world.

So why do we fall into a trap of constantly wishing for more? Is it because our society feeds us with lists of people who are each richer than the next? Why does that happen? Is it because it encourages us to strive and work harder, in order to earn more money to buy bigger and better things? Is it that, when someone has these things, we point at them and remark about how well that person has done when you only have blah blah blah… Thus the cycle continues, keeping us unhappy forever.

→ *Write your own definition*

If you're ready to break free from this cycle, and to start defining your own success, here's an easy tip: **DO NOT READ THOSE LISTS**. Forget how much money someone else has, and try not to define success by material possessions and wealth. When you move away from that, you can hopefully start to look at a person you care for and say, 'Well done, you've done it, I am proud of you,' without feeling jealous. You can be that person who holds hands rather than pushes them away. Be the person who celebrates your friends' good news and is genuinely happy for them, and who uses their excitement to spread their joy. It's much easier to do that if you're not desperately trying to achieve more than other people. If you are happy and spreading joy every day, that is the biggest measure of success.

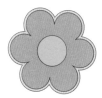

You are a success.

You're a *living, breathing* human being, and for that, you are *successful.*

THE ABILITY
TO SPREAD
JOY IS THERE
INSIDE OF
EACH OF US.

When people ask why I feel so strongly about spreading joy, I always reply with, 'Wouldn't this world be better if we spread

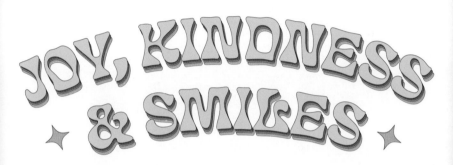

JOY, KINDNESS & SMILES

instead of constantly pushing for more?' That doesn't mean that we don't keep trying and learning, it just means that we really need to appreciate the moments that are happening now, not be constantly looking forward to tomorrow.

That little thing inside of you

I'd like to share a tale of the delivery driver. His name is Alex. He and I had a very long chat on the doorstep. He arrived playing some Aretha Franklin very loudly and was singing along to her song 'Respect'. I could hear him from inside whilst I was writing.

I opened the door and told him that he had a great voice and that he'd made me smile. He told me that he loved life and he'd always wanted to be a singer but he'd never had the breaks. He loved being a delivery driver because it permitted him to sing all day and meet different people and it enabled him to enjoy looking at life around him.

He told me he was in his forties and had never felt as content as he does now. Since he was a child, he had wanted nothing more than to bring people joy, and he'd always thought he would be able to do so through singing. I told him that even though he wasn't a professional singer, he was still bringing joy. He said a few people ask him to quieten down, but he just smiles and carries on singing. In my opinion, Alex has found that little thing inside of him that not only makes him happy, but makes others smile too.

Everyone has this little thing inside of them; for me, it is wanting to entertain others and make them happy. From the age of three years old, TV was – and still is – my dream, and little did I know that I would end up working in radio, too, which I also thoroughly enjoy because it's so personal. I honestly do know how unbelievably lucky I am to be following my dreams and to LOVE what I do.

→ *What's yours?*

What is the simplest thing that you love to do that could make someone smile today? If you enjoy connecting with others, it could be giving someone your total attention and time. When I was very little my mum would look for the same young woman at the checkout every week when we did our weekly supermarket shop, and she would chat to her for ages and ask her about her life. She was always so friendly and approachable and had a HUGE smile (as well as the longest ponytail I'd ever seen!), so maybe her little thing was connecting with others? Once you've identified that 'thing', know that it is your thing inside of you. And when you use it, you are making others happy and having a successful day, in my books.

Just in case you're wondering what happened to that checkout woman, I actually saw her a wee while ago walking down the street. She still had the longest ponytail, and when I saw her I smiled. She wouldn't have known why I smiled, but she smiled back, which immediately brought back memories of my late mum. These simple connections can still spread joy – even many years later.

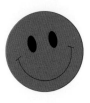

Surround yourself with good people

I have to be completely truthful with you, I didn't know I was going to write about friendship in this book. But when I started writing, I realised that friendship really is one of the most joyful things around. On the flipside, though, bad friends can result in sapping joy from us.

Many many years ago I worked on and off with some very negative people who spent a huge amount of their time gossiping and not being very nice. They were bullies and also very jealous of others. When you're in the midst of friendships like these — which, let's be honest, are quite toxic — it can be very difficult to NOT take these people's actions to heart. I'd like to share something I realised quite quickly while being around these people: when they are acting like this, and are being nasty to you, it's often because they're dealing with their own 'stuff' or they feel intimidated by you. In other words, they are behaving like this because of things to do with THEM and things going on in their own lives, not with YOU. It's a very difficult thing to remember, and even harder to take on board and to see, especially when someone that you consider to be a friend is acting this way, but they are probably sad and in turn are taking this out on others, rather than focusing on fixing themselves.

If your friends let you down, it is most probably not because of anything that you've done. Remembering this is so important, because this will help you to try to hold on to any joy and happiness. My late mum used to say to me, 'Keep your friends close but your enemies closer.' I have my own take on this: when people that you know are being horrible, be nice and kind to them whenever you can be. Because when you're kind, what can they then say back? Plus, you'll know in your heart that you've done all that you can despite how they've acted. You have attempted to make life easier and better for you all, and what's more, as these people probably need more joy in their life, maybe, just possibly, showing them kindness might help them.

→ *Be selective*

That being said, something that's hugely important to remember is that we have the power to pick our friends. And the older we get, the more we realise that we don't have to hold on to the friends who don't make us feel good, or who don't listen to us when we are down. So my best tip of all if you are experiencing any negative friendships that aren't bringing you joy, is to extricate yourself as soon as possible. I know this can be unbelievably difficult, and there are times where you can't do this – perhaps the friend in question works closely with you or is a family member who you simply can't avoid – but walking away when friendships are too toxic is a very powerful thing to do.

Break the toxic tie

Walking away shows strength – and we all have that inside of us. Walking away doesn't necessarily have to mean giving up on your friendship completely, it could just mean having a quick break or even just a walk outside, taking yourself out of the situation for a few moments, smiling, breathing and resetting. Restoring that joy in your soul.

If you have tried and tried to give this person joy and they simply cannot accept it, and it's hurting you to continue to spend time around them, then it is time to say goodbye and avoid any more pain. If you are going through this, remember to share how you feel with someone else. Talking always, ALWAYS helps. If you feel that you have no one to talk to, you'll find a list of amazing charities at the end of this book who are there for you to talk to when you need them.

→ *Be very selective*

We all have anxiety about our friends while we are growing up, asking ourselves all sorts of questions. Why don't I have as many friends as so-and-so? Why aren't I going out to wherever when the 'others' are? But over the years you come to understand why older people always say that you'll end up with fewer, but dearer, friends as you get older. I am very blessed to have some extremely special friends who I cannot thank enough for being there for me. They never fail to bring me joy. My best friend Celia has been by my side since we were 16; she's still my best friend and I couldn't wish for a better one. I have the most amazing group of gorgeous friends who I tell as often as I can that I love them. Some are new, some old, but all are so very dear to me and I know I am blessed to have them around me.

So, please do me a favour and think about who your friends are. Also consider, do they bring positivity into your life, or are they actually secretly quite toxic? You might not think it, but you really can break those ties. The friends who bring us joy are the ones we trust, the ones we know have our backs. Surround yourself with these people and consider why it is that you are friends with the others.

We all have choice. If you can keep those closest to you as good, positive forces, that will help you to *maintain joy* elsewhere. Don't just 'put up with' those people who never seem to care, never make you feel comfortable and who you can't be yourself with.

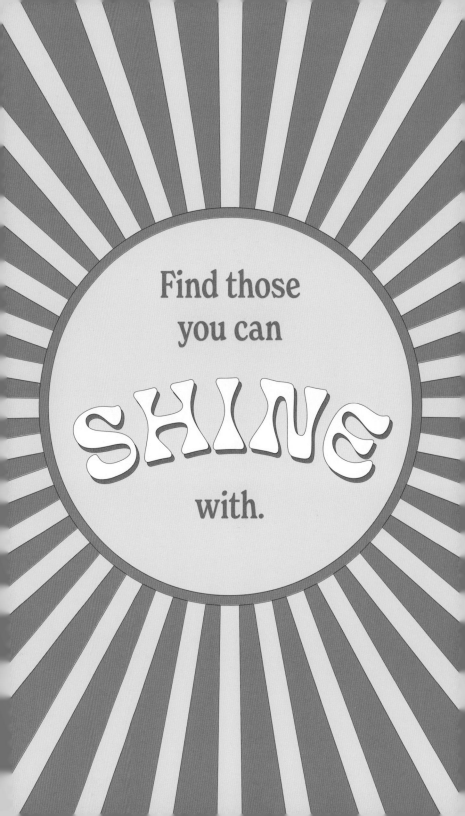

Find those
you can

SHINE

with.

Chapter

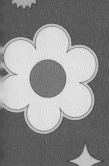

Ap
the Little

02

preciate
Things

When was the last time you stopped and looked at something when you were out walking? Or decided to take a stroll somewhere rather than choose the quickest way to get from A to B? When was the last time you bought yourself a little treat, or stopped to breathe in a huge lungful of a scent that you absolutely love? These are all little things that we can do so easily to feel more joy, but we often take them for granted. We rush when we walk, or we eat our treats really quickly, because we just need to do these things to get a fast 'feel-better fix' before we can start thinking about the next big worry in our lives.

In other words, we all spend so much time fretting about the big stuff that we forget to do the little things, but really appreciating the little things can be an incredible way of spreading joy. When I properly stop, take a breath and smile at the world around me, I feel lighter, brighter and more able to cope with the big stuff in my life – which is why I've dedicated an entire chapter to these things.

It wasn't until after I started walking everywhere (which I'll talk about a lot here, as it really has been so transformative for me) that I began to appreciate little things that many people might consider silly or inconvenient:

looking at the leaves

watching a squirrel running

listening to the wind in the trees

But now I stop and take in all of these things, and I feel so much better for it. At some point, I decided to start taking pictures, too, so that the joyful memories could last longer, then I post them to my Instagram, where people found that these pictures also helped them.

Little things lead to big things

These little things can bring more than just brief moments of joy, as I discovered recently when I pitched a huge TV project. I had a meeting in which I knew that my colleague and I would have to do the 'big sell', so I left home earlier than usual to give myself time to do one very little thing: I wanted to walk down some streets I'd never been down before, because I knew that this would enable me to look at the bigger picture, which I hoped would help me sort out the meeting in my mind, too. I was both nervous and excited in equal measure, and I needed some space in my head.

While I was out, I stopped to take a photo of a phone box. In doing so, a memory shot back to me. When I was fourteen, I phoned a boy that I fancied at school (his name was Adam) from a phone box so that he wouldn't know it was me and my parents wouldn't overhear me. He picked up the phone and instantly knew it was me and asked why I was calling. I told him that I liked him, and he made it clear that he wasn't interested in the slightest. The memory made me smile so much – calling Adam to tell him I liked him, now that took balls. At the time, I didn't give myself credit for what I'd done, and I probably wallowed for too long in my rejection, but standing there so many years later, looking at this phone box, this memory made me realise that I was so much stronger than I thought.

So I took my newfound resolve and started singing and skipping along to the meeting – I talked to people in the streets, I looked at the sun flickering through the trees in the park, and by the time I arrived I was in a very happy mood and felt ready to cope with the pitch. The meeting was full of laughter and joy, and when we left, I knew that taking those few moments to remove myself from the fear and worry, and to smile instead, had stopped me from fretting and helped the meeting to go well.

All the things that I'm going to discuss in this chapter are very simple. You will almost certainly have been told before how helpful they all are, but you might have forgotten over time. Equally, you might think that some of them are silly and too time-consuming when you have more important things to be doing. I'd like to reassure you here that even though they are simple, they will still hugely help you. Take this chapter as me giving you a gentle nudge to remind you just how important and how precious the simple things in life are.

(Oh, and if you're wondering about Adam, I actually bumped into him only a few years ago and he said he never knew I'd liked him at school. Oh yes he did!)

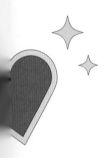

The power of positive thinking

Can you remember the last time you had a day in which everything seemed to go your way? Where you felt happy at nearly every moment, so much so that the day felt a little bit magical? I can almost guarantee that the day you're picturing in your mind is one you were really looking forward to, when you woke up and thought, 'Today is going to be brilliant.'

The odd thing, though, is that this brilliant day might have only been so brilliant because you woke up and decided that it would be.

Starting your day with a positive mindset makes it so much more likely that it will go well. We find this mindset very easy to adopt when we are about to enter a day that we have really been looking forward to, but much harder to do when it is full of less exciting things. In fact, on an average day, I'm sure that many people fall into a trap of imagining the worst things that could happen to them, or hundreds of 'what ifs?' before they have even got out of bed in the morning.

You don't need to do this.

We each have the power to reprogram how we think, and changing our own inner dialogue can be a very powerful way of having a much more joyful day.

Over the years, I have trained myself to step away from this negative narrative at the start of the day. Instead, I begin each day in a way that makes me feel happy: every single day for many years, the first thing I have done when I wake up is smile. I've been doing it for so long now that I do it subconsciously. I know that when you're feeling down and sad, smiling is extremely tough, so to help you, here's a bit of the sciencey stuff. Smiling keeps stress at bay; when you smile, your brain releases dopamine, endorphins and serotonin. All these things lower anxiety and increase the feeling of happiness.

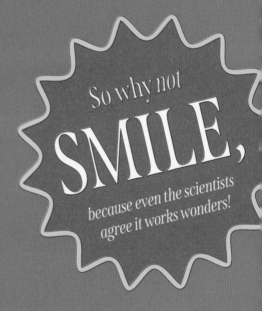

So why not **SMILE,** because even the scientists agree it works wonders!

Spread a smile

Give this a try. I'd like you to imagine that you're looking at someone sad, someone who is feeling broken. You decide to smile at them because you know that person will feel better if you do so, even for a moment, because someone cared enough to smile at them. That sad person is you sometimes. You need to smile at them to make them happier!

Be the person who spreads smiles. Even when I went through the crappiest of times, I continued to smile in the morning, and it did really set me up for the day. I passed this 'trick' on to a couple who I am very close to, who were dealing with something deeply personal in their lives. The wife called me up ten days later and said that the small smile had helped her – she had even ended up giggling most mornings (although I must admit that this was mainly because she found herself swearing at me for forcing her to smile). Smiling helps us to begin the day with a really positive mindset.

I start my day with a smile, then I like to take minute or so to think about the thing that I can't wait to happen in that day. Often this is something as simple as having a moment of laughter. And if I find that laughter isn't forthcoming, I try to make sure it happens through doing something that I really enjoy. I have found that smiling and having something to look forward to make my days just that little bit better.

I'd also really like to encourage you to take this positive mindset with you once you get out of bed. I'm not saying that you need to put a positive spin on everything to make it seem wonderful, or to look at yourself in the mirror and start saying, 'I am beautiful and today is going to be great.' If that's what helps you, though, please keep doing it. But what I'm asking you to do, rather than saying, 'What if?' is to try to say to yourself, 'I know today will have at least one great moment.' And instead of thinking 'I look crap today' or 'Don't I look tired?', try to think about how you feel: 'I feel okay today, I'm alright.' There we go, it's that simple.

Starting to think in a positive way and make yourself look forward to one little moment in the day that will make everything feel worthwhile means that joy will likely start to be more forthcoming.

Today's Tiny Tasks

1

Smile when you first wake up in the morning. Literally in that very moment, pop a smile on your face, and it will help you start your day with a brighter outlook. Try this every day for two weeks.

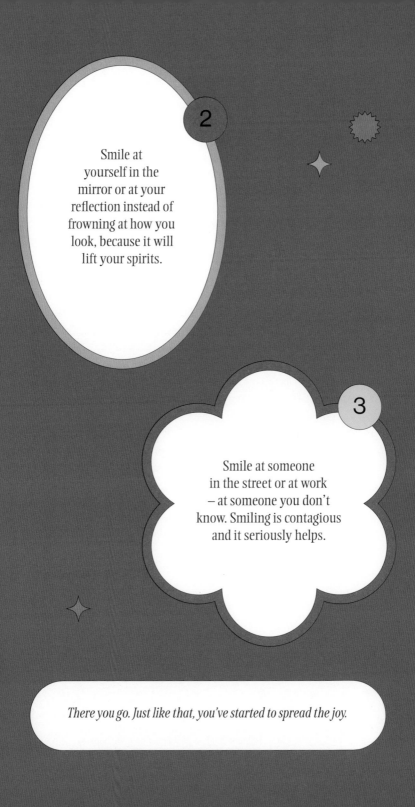

2

Smile at yourself in the mirror or at your reflection instead of frowning at how you look, because it will lift your spirits.

3

Smile at someone in the street or at work – at someone you don't know. Smiling is contagious and it seriously helps.

There you go. Just like that, you've started to spread the joy.

Make your *own* weather

Ever since I was very little I have been a sunshine lover. I don't mean one of the getting-a-tan-and-sitting-around-doing-nothing types of sunshine lover (although these days I fake tan it every day. Yes, I am loud and proud about my fake tan love.) No, I mean the type of person whose mood seems to be based on the weather. When I was a child, if the sun was out I would be super excited to get outside, but if it was raining, I'd be a grump. I would moan and ask how long the rain was going to last for. Of course, in those days we didn't have a minute-by-minute account of how the weather would change; we had one weather report, once a day, and if my mum couldn't remember when it said it would stop raining (and let's be honest, even if she could, it would usually be wrong), I would sit by the window watching the sky, ever hopeful that the grey skies would turn to blue and it would be sunny again soon.

Today, I am still as reliant upon the sun for an instant mood boost as I was then. This isn't something that's unique to me; doctors have been talking about SAD (Seasonal Affective Disorder) for many years now. In fact, for a long time when I spoke about the effect that the sun had on me, people would ask if I had SAD. I used to think I did, and I bought a special sunshine lamp to make it better, but I never used it (although I know many people who continue to swear by these, so if you do feel a little gloomy in the winter, looking into a SAD lamp might be a good idea). Instead, I started to rethink the way I thought about the weather and learnt much cheaper ways to bring sunshine into those rainy days.

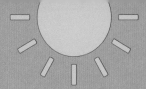

→ *Seek out light*

When we are in the darkest days (literally and emotionally), very often what we crave is light. So on those days, instead of thinking 'I wish it would be sunny,' I look at photos of sunshine and think to myself 'How lovely', imagining what a day of sun will look like, and I smile. Whenever there is even a teeny weeny bit of blue sky I will also squint my eyes and imagine the whole sky is blue. I know this sounds small and perhaps a bit silly, but it really helps. Once again, there is science behind this thought: researchers from the University of Sussex said that exposing yourself to the colour blue 'sent self-confidence soaring, cut stress and boosted happiness' and their study concluded that 'when people saw blue their brainwaves showed increased happiness'. The sky really is powerful!

Evoking the weather that makes you happiest doesn't just need to apply to those of us who like the sunniest of days – I realise that there are some people who don't! We have a dear friend who really dislikes the sunshine; darker wintery days make her happy. If that's what lifts your spirits too, why not try to imagine the days that you like best when the weather isn't what you want it to be? We don't have to settle for what we're given.

My final tip is that when the weather that you want to see materialises, make the most of it. The sun shone brightly this morning and I jumped out of bed (after my wake-up smile) and skipped to the bathroom. Ten minutes later the clouds appeared, but I held on to that feeling and decided not to let it disappear. It kept me smiling for most of the day.

Walking in the fresh air

I cannot tell you how much walking has given me. I am actually walking as I write this (well… recording it into my phone to write up later). Up until a few years ago, when my husband bought me a Fitbit watch (I do love a bit of tech!), walking was something that I did very rarely. When I first got my fitness watch I loved that I now had a way to count my steps, and I wondered how many miles I did in a day. That's where it all began – and those who follow me on Instagram or listen to my various shows will know that I now walk EVERYWHERE, and if I don't walk I don't feel as good.

I started by seeing how many steps I could fit into a day around my routine. I didn't start by walking miles, I just decided to walk to the next tube station instead of jumping on at our local stop. I quickly grew to love the feeling of elation that not taking the easy option gave me and I started to get excited about the distance I was covering. Each week I slowly started to build up my steps, and I couldn't quite believe it when they were amounting to 3 miles' worth of walking, then 4, and so on. I remember walking 5 miles and ringing my husband because I couldn't believe that I could get so much done. I felt so much happier and energised. Now, when I don't walk, I feel smaller – yep, at 5 foot 8 and three-quarters that may not make sense, but walking makes me feel taller. Sensing the ground beneath my feet makes me feel rooted, and that, in turn, makes me feel more confident and happier in myself.

Walking also helps me open my mind, my heart and my ears. It feeds my fascination for knowing what's going on around me. Too many of us spend our time with our heads looking downwards. We so rarely look up and around at our surroundings, and what we are missing is too valuable.

My mum spent years trying to teach me this; she would go on and on about taking our dog Bazooka (a glorious Staffordshire bull terrier) out for a walk. I enjoyed those walks, but I didn't get excited by them like I do about my walks now. For years afterwards I'd jump in the car, or on the tube, bus or train instead of walking. I'd go to the gym to exercise but I would take the car to get there. I'd walk when on holiday to see the sights, but back home the only time I'd see the sights would be if I was carried there on wheels. Everything was 'quicker' that way, and I'd also get everywhere without ever looking windswept. But in getting everywhere faster, I didn't realise that I was missing out on so many of the beautiful things that the world has to offer.

How that has all changed! Walking didn't enter my realm for a long time, but now that it has, what it's done for my mind, body and soul has been remarkable. Because of walking, my mind is less frenetic. As someone who finds it hard to stop thinking, walking calms me and allows me to have more organised thoughts, which has been a joyous gift. What's even more interesting is that walking also makes me feel more focused. My ideas are more honed after I've walked. It's not that my mind switches off when walking, it just switches on in a new way. I see things on a bigger scale; I'm able to streamline my thoughts, and ideas seem to pop up from nowhere.

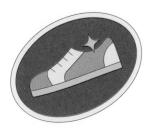

There have been so many studies to show the great value that walking brings to us, and we now know that it is great for your body. If you're able to walk, just getting up and moving means your blood is pumping and your muscles are moving, and you are more than likely feeling better as well. It reduces the risk of heart disease and strokes. It's good for lowering high blood pressure. It can help to make your bones stronger and relieve joint pain and stiffness. In other words, it's really, really good for you.

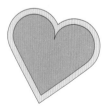

WALKING

helps me
open my

MIND,

my

HEART

and my

EARS.

Sensing the GROUND beneath my feet makes me feel ROOTED, and that, in turn, makes me feel MORE confident and HAPPIER in myself.

→ *Make your journey joyful*

You may be wondering how walking will help you spread the joy, though. Well, it's simple. If we feel more joyful, we will start to pass on those joyful feelings to others. When I walk to a destination, I arrive happier. And when I'm happy I tend to see my happiness rubbing off onto others. I am elated by what I've seen and heard when I'm walking, as well as by my body moving. It also gives me the space I need to 'feel' my emotions; something that we are all very quick to block, because 'not' feeling them can be easier to handle. We are, bizarrely, taught to do this in order to be strong. I have fallen victim to this, too; I remember saying to my best friend at my mum's funeral, 'Don't hug me or be nice because then I'll break, and I need to be strong for Dad.' This is such a natural reaction for people to have in difficult situations, but it's not a good way to be. Those feelings of happiness or sadness need to be allowed out. I can tell you that I am far better at listening to my emotions now. If I am sad I talk about what's making me sad, and I let myself feel that way. Not for long, I must admit, because I am someone who lives in the moment, and agonising over events that make you sad can stop you from doing this. And when I feel happy, I want to share that too.

> Instead of being strong, how about just being you? Give yourself that space to feel.

Now, I completely understand that some people might be indifferent about walking, and that others might feel terrified by the concept. You might be worried that you won't be able to walk 'far enough' or that you'll get bored. Regardless of how you feel about walking right now, I'd like you to set yourself a challenge: leave your home, walk to the end of your road and count how many steps it takes you to get there. You might be surprised by how far it is! Then walk back, but this time don't count your steps; just have a look around. What do you see? Here's the thing: this might seem like a very little push right now, but a little push can become a lot in a very short space of time.

Let me tell you a story about my dad; he is in his late eighties now but he walks at least a mile and a half a day. He started during lockdown when I was worried about him being alone in his house (as so many of us did about our relatives and friends), so I kept on at him to walk. He said he couldn't, so I told him to use the step counter on his mobile to measure how far he could go just around his sitting room and in his garden. He spoke to me every day and would say how he was amazed by how far he'd walked in just 30 minutes. It gave him purpose across the long days where we had nothing else to do, kept him fit and gave him something to talk about.

Dad still walks, but now he goes outside into the streets and parks local to him. He uses a stick (which he really didn't want to accept that he needed at first but is now obsessed with) to manage his daily walks, and all this has done the world of good for his body and mental health. If a walk is all he does in one day, he still feels he's accomplished something when he tells us how far he's managed. He has seen the world going on around him and he feels a sense of joy. I must be honest, he's still not one for walking out in the rain, but that's understandable at his age.

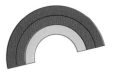

Banish worries

Do you feel worried about walking? Ask yourself, what is it that you're scared of? Sometimes you just need someone to ask you what the fear is before you can become aware of it yourself. A few people have told me that they're worried about needing the loo on a long walk. If this is you, I would like you to put those fears out of your mind. When I walk, I ask cafes and restaurants if I can please use their facilities, and nobody has ever said no. Maybe you're afraid you'll be late to your destination, but guess what, now that I walk everywhere, I am always on time. This is because I can more accurately judge the time when I need to leave, because I know how long the walk will take me. I'm not at the beck and call of bus or train timetables or traffic jams.

The other question I often get is how I manage to look okay when I arrive at work or to a meeting when I've walked there. Here's the thing – I simply tell people that I walked. I am proud of being a walker. I often have messed-up hair when I arrive, and I just don't care. I have also embraced the trainers way of life. Take it from an obsessive heel wearer who believed that giving in to flats never was an option – goodness me, I was missing a lot before. Mainly, the ability to walk for long distances, of course!

→ *Walking is a gift*

When the Queen died last year, many of us felt an unbelievable sense of loss. In the days leading up to her state funeral, along with many thousand others, I went to Buckingham Palace to pay my quiet respects. I remember walking there and when I arrived at Green Park I was overwhelmed by the sweet smell of flowers and the feeling of love and calm. I stood and looked at the flowers, smiled and had a tear in my eye at some of the messages. I then walked on to the palace, where I smiled and chatted to some wonderful people from the UK, along with many tourists too.

When I crossed the road to leave, I saw a tall young volunteer gently hugging a very elderly woman. He looked at me and mouthed that she was sobbing. I gently touched her arm and asked if I could help. One of the lovely things about being on the telly for many years is people know me and are happy to chat. She wiped her eyes and said, 'Hello Gaby'. I asked if she wanted to go for a cup of tea and she said she'd like to sit and talk to me for a while, so we did just that. She took a beautiful card out of her bag which she said was one of her most treasured possessions. It was a card from the Queen that had been sent to her on the occasion of her 60th wedding anniversary in 2019. She opened it up and asked me to read it. After I'd finished, she said, 'That's me, Iris, and that was my husband.' She told me that he had sadly passed away just a couple of months after their anniversary. She said she loved the Queen and was so devastated by her death that she felt compelled to come to the palace every single day until her funeral. She then said that she walked there and back each day and that walking was her most favourite thing. She was in her late eighties and she was walking over 8 miles a day to visit Buckingham Palace! I spent a while with her and totally fell for her. We laughed together and talked about her life. When she walked off waving goodbye, she told me that if there was any life lesson to teach it was to walk everywhere. She said, 'It'll keep you young. Your body and your mind will thank you.' I will never forget Iris and I am passing on her advice to you all: KEEP WALKING if you possibly can!

keep WALK- ING

if you possibly can!

Today's Tiny Tasks

1

Walk to the end of your street and count how many steps it takes. When you get there, just turn around and walk back home, but this time look around you. When you get in, add up your steps (just double your outward-bound step count).

2

Park the car further away
from home and work – this
way you're forced to do
some walking.

3

If you're travelling by public transport,
get off a stop earlier than you would do usually. It
really is that simple. Yes, it may add a few minutes to
your journey, but what you've now gained in doing
all these Tiny Tasks is huge.

*And this is an important note for this Task: tell everyone you
possibly can that you're walking more and see their reaction; nine
out of ten of them will congratulate you, and the one who doesn't say
anything will be the person who you need to help on their walking
journey. Yes, they'll growl and groan and say they can't, but they
can. And in getting them walking, you can help spread the joy.*

The importance *of* looking

I decided to set myself a challenge: I had to look at something I was doing that would ordinarily annoy me for at least a few minutes before I could lift my eyes away. We often have to do this when we try to untie a shoelace that's knotted, or we can't untwist the wires of our headphones, and I think anyone would struggle to not find these moments frustrating. But I'm not talking about these things, I'm talking about the times when you might look at a pile of washing-up that you asked someone to do but they haven't, or the bed that you had intended to make in the morning but never got round to, or the puddle you've just accidentally stepped in that's made your shoes all wet. When do we look at something like this, something that might be considered a little mundane and frustrating, for more than just a few seconds? Probably never, especially if you're like me and attempting to do a few things at once. When I started practising this, I was surprised to find that, over the course of a few minutes, my frustration started to slip away and my imagination would run wild instead.

The first time I tried this out, I'd gone to the sink to pour myself a glass of water and found coffee grounds at the bottom of it. My husband religiously has two cups of coffee every day (I don't drink coffee at all) and always leaves some grounds in the sink. When I saw them, instead of growling about the fact he'd done this again, I paused. I looked at the pattern they made and decided it looked like a duck. I called him over to look at the duck. He couldn't see it at all to start off with, but when I asked him to 'just look' he said he could maybe see a sort of duck (ish), which we both laughed at. I pointed out that we'd just shared joy together, to which he replied, 'Don't be daft, that's just you trying to look on the bright side.' Maybe that's true and I am just trying to look on the bright side, but wouldn't it be nicer if we could all do that more often, rather than feeling annoyed?

I know this may sound a little crazy, but trust me on this, and if you want to try it, here's a sort of checklist of things to look out for when you are walking.

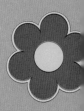

Feel the joy

1

Notice the leaves on the trees. That sounds simple, but remember that each leaf is unique – no two leaves are ever identical. My dear friend told me this at a moment that I needed to hear it. Now I will never forget it and it's such a magical fact.

2

Look for colour around you. You will see it even on the greyest of days; it may not come along as a flower in midwinter, but buildings have colour, people wear colour (especially if they read this book!). There's colour everywhere, just take a moment to look for it.

3

See someone smiling. Yes, believe it or not many people smile; if you spot someone smiling, try sending a smile back.

4

Take note of delivery drivers singing, postmen whistling, street cleaners dancing, children skipping (go on, try a skip, because that does most definitely make you smile), postboxes with knitted hats on (yes, I keep spotting them around), window cleaners high up on tall buildings, and take a moment to feel the joy at your fingertips.

5

Spot birds in the trees, or simply pets trotting along.

All of these things are VERY simple and obvious. They are wonderful, they're free, and they're there for us all if we just take time to look. They may seem so obvious that you may possibly pooh pooh this list, and if you do, that's completely fine, but why not make your own list of things to look out for? Give it a go and pass your list on to others to see if they are really looking around too.

_____

_____

_____

_____

_____

_____

_____

_____

_____

_____

_____

_____

_____

_____

Adults often claim the world becomes less full of

MAGIC

as we get older, but this simply isn't true - we just don't allow ourselves the time to see it.

→ *Looking up*

If you take anything from this section (as well as the fact that walking is one of life's best gifts), it's that looking up is so important. We all spend so long on our phones or at our computers or watching TV – all of which I love to do (especially the TV part), so I am not judging you here – rather than looking at our surroundings, and this habit that we've developed is causing us to live in a bubble. When you truly open your eyes, you'll be amazed at what you'll see.

I know this sounds trite, but trust me. I'd forgotten that buildings had amazing architecture, or that birds sat in trees, or that the clouds made patterns in the sky. Aren't all those things magical? We all notice those things as children, but as adults we almost seem to lose the ability to do so. I remember playing the 'what can you see in that cloud?' game. How many of you still do this now? And if you don't, why don't you? Or the 'look, that tree has a face' game. I know you know the one… These things brought us so much joy when we were younger, but they aren't games just for children, they haven't gone away or left you, and you shouldn't feel as though you aren't able to see them again. Adults often claim the world becomes less full of magic as we get older, but this simply isn't true – we just don't allow ourselves the time to see it. Walking opens your eyes once more and lets you see the world as it's supposed to be, full of wonder.

Use your nose

Here's a strange thing that I'd like to share: I could never ever smell things when I was young. In fact, I was constantly blocked up and nasal. I didn't know at the time, but a food allergy was the cause of all of that congestion, which I only found out about when I was in my early twenties. Once I was diagnosed and managed to cut that specific food out of my diet, I could suddenly breathe properly and also smell so many things for the very first time.

Now, with my food allergy under control, I have a super-nose. No, my nose doesn't wear a cape and fly around saving the universe, AND I don't mean I love the look of my nose or that it's particularly big – what I mean is I can now smell everything very strongly. This is absolutely brilliant, because I love smells – they are so evocative. I can always be found sniffing flowers, walking into bakeries and breathing in a good old lungful of the heady bready smells (which is ironic, to be honest, as I have a proper allergy to gluten and wheat), and when I arrive on holiday I always go on about the 'hot holiday place smell'. All of these aromas make me feel incredibly warm and happy inside.

So, I would love to encourage you to open up your minds and of course your nostrils to the scents around you. Sniff that pink rose in your friend's front garden. Take a deep inhale when you get onto public transport – yes, sometimes the smells might not be pleasant, but breathing in will really help you to be in the moment and notice the things around you. Your head is out of your phone and your olfactory senses are going through that Rolodex in your brain, and, you never know, maybe some memories will also suddenly reappear. One of my absolute favourite smells is that of the perfume my fantastic Granny Moo (her name was Muriel, so her nickname was Moo) wore. She died in 1999 and I still miss her so much, but whenever I get a whiff of her perfume on a passer-by, I breathe in her smell and smile hugely. I definitely had the best Granny on the planet.

IF WE DON'T ALLOW OURSELVES SOME *SIMPLE TREATS*, LIFE JUST GETS *DOWNRIGHT TOUGH*.

Treat yourself

For me, the best treat has always been ice cream. This goes right back to my childhood. I remember visiting a lovely family-run Italian gelato place that was close to our house when I was a little girl. It was slightly out of the way – we didn't pass it if we were heading anywhere like the shops, or to school – so if we ever started driving in its direction, we would all cheer loudly because we knew that we were heading for ice cream. If we were all together as a family, my mum probably would have had to have been persuaded to join us on our ice cream jaunt by my dad. She wasn't a fan. Me and my dad, though, have always shared our love for ice cream.

I would always have the same flavour – strawberry. I would be allowed two scoops and would eat it far too quickly and get brain freeze. (In fact, I still do that… note to self, must eat slower.) When we went away on our family holidays abroad, I would sometimes really rock the boat and combine a scoop of strawberry with a scoop of banana. I still love that combination now, although my favourite flavour nowadays is definitely pistachio. Isn't it funny how our taste buds change over the years? If someone had told me that I would have loved (and, trust me, it really is a love!) a green nutty ice cream when I was a child, I would have told them they were mad and made one of those 'that's yucky' faces. But I have gone to the pistachio side now and there really is no turning back.

It was this passion that made me decide on a cold, rainy and windy day by the beach in Cornwall recently, when I was feeling a little gloomy, that I would love an ice cream. So I bought one. The strange looks I got were so funny – I was even asked if I really wanted one. I smiled and nodded and explained to the very friendly woman serving me that I loved ice cream and I didn't care about the weather; ice cream isn't just for sunny days, but for life. She giggled and gave me a massive scoop or two in a tub. I did think how bizarre it was that I was being questioned whether I was really sure. I knew I needed a treat and buying myself an ice cream made me feel so much joy.

I am passionate about health and fitness and have spent many, many years researching and studying health (ever since my father was diagnosed with bowel cancer in 1996). I know that what we eat is vitally important, and that generally, ice cream isn't one of the foods that's considered to be very 'healthy'. (I know. I'm sad too.) But here's the thing. I love ice cream, and I believe that my love for it is healthy; and that's because I am a strong believer that the foods that we love are huge treats to have in moderation, of course, but can also bring us joy.

We all need to give ourselves a treat every so often. For many people that might be chocolate, but I need to come clean now and tell you that I don't like chocolate. Never have. Yes, I know you think I'm mad, but I think it tastes yukky. I live in a family of chocolate lovers, but it really isn't for me, thank you very much. You can keep your chocolate bars and mini eggs.

→ Grown-ups need treats too

When we were younger, we may all have been lucky enough to have someone in our circle who would give us treats; an adult who might take us out to the park, or make us a lovely dinner, or buy us some chocolate (despite that not being my idea of a treat). As adults, though, we might not have someone who is specifically looking out to treat us and we are often so wary of treating ourselves – thinking that it shows some sort of weakness of character or makes us look selfish; a chink in our adult armour.

But treats are vital for bringing joy when we're feeling low! It doesn't have to be something big – in fact, it's my opinion that the best ones are often small. It could be ice cream (of course!), or a bath, or a moment that you spend watching an old YouTube clip, or maybe even just having that second piece of buttery toast. If we don't allow ourselves some simple treats, life just gets downright tough.

We must be gentler on ourselves. How about making yourself a list of all the little treats that bring you happiness, or picking your favourite treat (like I have) and using it to bring joy on a rainy day? Just remember, the word 'treat' literally means 'an event or item that is out of the ordinary and gives great pleasure', so we can't use treats to feel good all the time, otherwise their effects wear off. For long-term joy, we need of course to dig a little deeper…

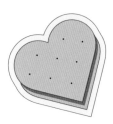

Joyful foods

So many of our favourite tastes come from memories; ice cream is likely my favourite treat because of the wonderful times that I had of eating it with my family as a child.

What foods are associated with the memories that you hold dear? These can be used as a pick-me-up when you need a little boost. If none come to mind, why not create some joyful memories with food now? Find those things that you like to eat and take special people with you that you'd like to eat them with. I know this may sound a bit daft and odd, but this is laying down your future memories.

And remember, if you want to have some ice cream, do it. It doesn't matter if it's rainy or cold or cloudy. Let's not judge when one of the best foods on the planet should be eaten.

Chapter_

You_____

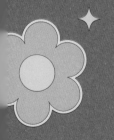

*the_*

03

_Make
___Rules

There is some
sort of
unwritten
rule in society
that as soon
as we hit a
certain age,

the magic of
the world needs
to fade, and
with it our

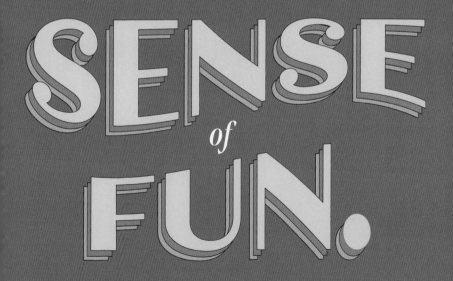

SENSE *of* FUN.

When someone says that someone should 'act like they are a grown-up', what do they mean? There is some sort of unwritten rule in society that as soon as we hit a certain age, the magic of the world needs to fade, and with it our sense of fun. Once we reach adulthood, we are suddenly supposed to conceal our emotions; it seems we can't sit and daydream, and we certainly can't wear things that are bright and fun and colourful.

If we say that we want to do something spontaneous and silly, we're told to not be daft – we have responsibilities and we need to go and fulfil them while being really serious. Of course, I know that with adulthood come more responsibilities – and we do need to cope with the harsh realities of paying bills, filling out forms, going to work and completing other important chores – but that doesn't mean you can't have an immense amount of fun along the way.

The sad thing is, though, that because many of us fear being judged, we often go through our adult lives doing the things that are expected of us, in the way that we are told to do them. We do these things so often that these unwritten societal rules begin to feel as if they are part of our personalities – and not one of them makes us feel more joyful.

These rules drive me mad – I get most angry when I see headlines in magazines, papers or online articles that read: 'Once you're over a certain age you shouldn't…', which is then followed by a whole list of things that I should no longer be allowed to do 'at my age'. How dare they tell me not to have long hair or wear shorter skirts? I honestly want to tell them to sod off, because I don't want to be told how to be.

> Doing things that society considers daft does make me more happy, so I don't want to stop doing them purely because I am getting older.

In this chapter, I'm going to explain why it is that I think it's time that we stop following the so-called rules, why it is that we should all be aiming to release our inner child a little more, and I'm going to help you make up your own rules. We'll be speaking about how, if something makes you happy, you should do it. How, if your friend wants to do something that he has never done before (if it's safe to do so and won't hurt anyone in the process), then we should not tell him he can't. Let him give it a go. We don't have to behave like we are supposed to.

> As long as we are being kind, polite and trying to spread joy, we can do whatever we want – within reason.

The other rules that I'm going to be talking about breaking in this section are the ones we have made for ourselves; those that tell us we can't say no to something we don't want to do, that we can't break free from our daily routine, or that tell us we're too anxious to go and make a new friend. In this chapter, it really is time to remind yourself that you are able to do the things that you previously believed you couldn't – and find so much joy in the process. I know that fear can get in the way of this, but it's time to say bye-bye to that fear! I will be with you every step of the way.

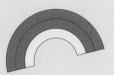

Releasing *your* inner child

I wonder when it is that we close that box – when it is that we say a silent goodbye to our inner child? I'm not sure exactly when it happened to me, but I do remember starting to think I had to be a 'grown up', and pretending to like coffee because that was 'cool' and 'adulty'. I remember saying that anything Disney was pathetic. But there have always been elements from my childhood that I've held on to. When everyone else was acting cool as a teenager, I would still be the one who would roll on my side down a hill or pretend I was hosting a TV show in my bedroom. (If YouTube had been around when I was younger I probably would have been creating content – but it wasn't, so all I had was the power of my imagination.) Some people would tell me that it was 'so uncool' for me to be doing these things, and while I didn't like hearing that at all because I was so self-conscious, I carried on because I knew that they made me so happy.

Jumping in puddles is something that every child loves to do; when I was little, there was nothing simpler than splashing about with my wellies on. I'm sure it was the same for you too. So why is it that we abandon these childhood pleasures when we grow up? What stops us from doing them? I think it's purely embarrassment, or a feeling of self-consciousness, or a tendency to forget to let the inner child in us out. We spend so much of our time worrying about what others think that we miss out on the simplest of joys.

Today, I continue to have fun and prioritise my inner child as much as I can. I still jump in puddles, and every time I do, I smile. I no longer get upset if people tell me that doing so is uncool. The child is there inside all of us, and I am giving you full permission to let it out again. We only live this life once – it's short and it's precious and the most fun times can be had when we prioritise innocent and simple fun. When your inner child is next screaming at you to throw that snowball, roll down that hill or play that game – let go of your inhibitions and do it!

Abandon your insecurities – take it from someone who held on to them for too long and is still shy at times, let out your inner child. It's the simple things that work when it comes to feeling joy.

Feel your emotions

There is nothing worse than bottling up your emotions – have you ever desperately tried to stop crying when you know the tears are threatening to come? It's so unbelievably difficult. And yet, in the UK, we are taught to be stoic (in other words, to be someone who can cope with hardship without showing their feelings). I'm sure that this has been part of a larger attempt to make the British feel brave and strong, but in all honesty, on a very human level, I have no idea why we were or continue to be taught this. Why shouldn't we show and feel things? Keeping them concealed can result in our emotions eating away at us from the inside and stifling any sense of joy.

I would consequently really like to encourage you, if you are feeling down, to not try to pack those feelings into a box in your mind. You don't need to wallow in your feelings, but you should acknowledge that you're feeling them. Let them wash over you; if this means you cry, so what? Crying can be cathartic sometimes. So, go ahead and break the rules you have been told about concealing your emotions and instead talk, share and discuss how you feel. You can do this with anyone – it doesn't need to be a friend or family member, as long as it is someone you trust.

Talking honestly will help, but if you're not in a place where you're able to do this yet, another option that helps so, so many people is writing down how you feel. When you do this, it can feel like you're being self-indulgent, but trust me when I say that you're not. I remember being very fed up with something that a newspaper had written about me because it wasn't true at all, and my friend advised me to write on a piece of paper how I felt, then screw it up and chuck it in a bin, as if I was chucking away the lies they'd written. I felt so much better when I had done just that. Simply writing your thoughts down on a scrap of paper to acknowledge how you are feeling can help you come to terms with that emotion enormously and, if it's a negative one, move on from it.

→ *Like and share*

On the flip side, when you feel happy, please make sure you
take a moment to sit with this emotion – and share it! Let others
know. There is a strange thing going around where people think
that it's 'unfair' to let others know if you're happy in case
they're not. Trust me when I say that when someone feels joy
radiating from you, they'll struggle to not feel a little happier
too. And being someone who helps others feel a bit better
is a gift that we need to share.

_____

_____

_____

_____

_____

_____

_____

_____

_____

_____

_____

Today's Tiny Tasks

1

On day one, try this: get a pen and a piece of paper and write down how you feel at this moment – just one word to describe your emotions. Write down any happy words, too, if you're feeling them!

2

The next day, write a whole sentence that describes how you feel. It doesn't have to be a work of great literature, oh no – it can simply say something along the lines of 'Today I feel a bit crap because I didn't hear from that person I wanted to get a text from,' or 'Today I feel great because I ate an orange and I like oranges.'

3

On day three, write more than one sentence about how you're feeling today, then read it out loud to yourself. Then look back to day one and re-read what you've written. Comparing how you feel from day to day will help you to focus in on the bigger picture, because suddenly the problems that you had before will likely start to feel small now they are in the past.

#Shoppinginyourwardrobe

A few years ago, I started something on my Instagram that has grown much bigger than I ever imagined. I call it #Shoppinginyourwardobe. Originally it was a kind of fingers up at the influencers who posed in expensive clothes to encourage us to buy what they were wearing. I got annoyed when I tapped on something and loved it but couldn't afford it. But then I would look in my own wardrobe and realise I had something similar that I had bought years ago, and I didn't need a new thing at all. Fashion trends get recycled time and time again, so you might be surprised to discover that the same thing will probably happen to you, too.

So, I popped on a couple of things that I had never worn together before and my youngest daughter took a photo. I then decided it would be even funnier if I made a video and sang a very annoying song – the now-infamous 'shopping in your wardrobe' jingle. I then continued to grab things out of my cupboards, or my daughters' or my husband's (although a little disclaimer here, you may want to check with your family before walking downstairs in their clothes…!), and wore them as I had never worn them before. Not only did I really enjoy this, when I posted it on my Instagram, everyone else seemed to love it too: the song gradually started to be sung in other people's videos on social media. There is immense pressure for people to be constantly buying new things nowadays to slot into the latest trends – especially on social media – and I think everyone was quite happy that there was someone on this platform saying you don't need to rush out and spend money you don't have.

I've always been an advocate for finding different ways to feel cool that don't cost the earth. When I was fifteen I worked in a local shop that sold papers, magazines, vinyls and small gifts. I worked there every single Saturday and Sunday for many years before I headed off to college (and loved it); in my lunch break on a Saturday I would sometimes go to the local street market. I couldn't afford to buy clothes from brands that everyone was wearing (at the time, it was original Levi's), so I would buy imitations of them. I was proud when I managed to find jeans that looked just like the labels I wanted to wear, and I used to tell everyone that they were bargains from the market. One girl would always look down her nose at me, but that didn't stop me. I didn't want to spend time worrying about what other people thought of me.

I truly believe that shopping in your wardrobe (silly song optional) spreads so much joy. It's so easy to do, and the benefits go beyond the cost to your purse. I learnt a few years ago how hugely damaging the fast-fashion industry is to our planet, and shopping in your wardrobe enables us to do our bit to start moving away from purchasing new clothes that align with seasonal trends. Yes, I know many people don't feel confident to do this because they're worried that they'll be judged for wearing older clothes, but please just try. So many people are proudly wearing outfits from vintage stores and charity shops these days. No one is judging you and PLEASE don't judge yourself!

Start simply. Look at your clothes. Now really look. Stand back and ignore all of your usual favourites. Those black jeans that you wore for all of last week? No, not getting your attention. Your favourite jumper? Definitely not! Look for those items you haven't worn for a while or that you wish you were still young enough to wear (trust me, you are!). Grab literally anything that you haven't worn in a long time. Maybe it's an old top that you convinced yourself not to give away because you'd wear again, but that hasn't seen the light of day in years. Now put it on. Only now are you allowed to go back and find that favourite pair of trousers or jacket and pop it on too. Not only do you look great in a whole new outfit that you've probably never worn before, you haven't spent a penny and the planet is happier. It's a joyful win-win.

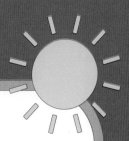

Stuff the rules

If you want to take it to the next level, why not create a drop? What's that, I hear you cry. Well, it's a DRess that you're wearing as a tOP. No sewing involved (phew, eh?). With a 'drop', that old dress that may be too short or a summer dress that you want to wear on chillier days can still be worn regularly. Take some looser-fitting jeans or trousers or skirt, tuck the dress in or use a belt to keep the bottom up, and now you're wearing it as a top. I do this often. It brings a whole new life to older items in your wardrobe.

Speaking of summer clothes, why not pop a jumper or sweatshirt over a summer dress? For some stupid reason, I never used to wear my summer outfits in the winter. What a total waste of money that was! There are ways around the lighter material that summer clothes are made out of. I have a lovely white dress with black dots all over it, but it's made from the lightest material; I also have an old, white, long-sleeved, thermal T-shirt, which I now wear underneath this dress. And with black boots as well, it works perfectly at any time of year. So why not wear your summer outfits all year round? Stuff the rules.

The importance *of* spontaneity

Breaking away from your daily routine can bring you endless amounts of joy; there really is nothing simpler to make you happy than doing something unexpected. Surprises can be so thrilling (for my dad, for example, there's nothing better than a friend of his appearing unexpectedly, or us saying we are popping round with not much notice); yet we are all so ruled by our calendars, by the routines that we have built up for ourselves, that often unplanned or new things can initially feel difficult to slot in. Then before long, we become scared of doing something new altogether – which utterly fascinates me. When we are kids we have our routines, but around that, we try new tastes and activities all the time. We may be slightly wary of them, but we usually give it a go. At what age does this start to change? And why?

The ability to be spontaneous is something that you probably don't think about much, because of the general busy-ness of life. Right now, though, I would like you to pause and think about the last time that you did something on a whim. If you can't remember when you last did something you hadn't planned, ask yourself why that is. Take a moment to think about why it is that you feel you can't be spontaneous.

I decided to ask a few people this exact question, and here are their responses:

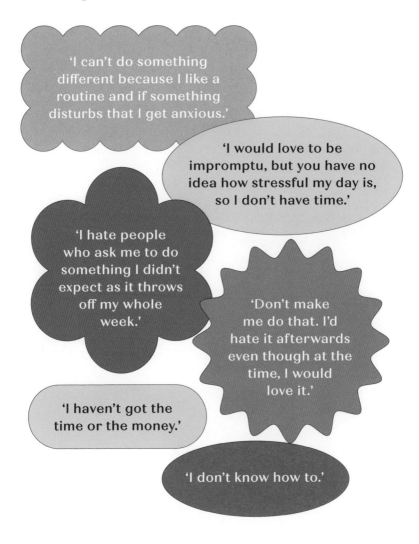

'I can't do something different because I like a routine and if something disturbs that I get anxious.'

'I would love to be impromptu, but you have no idea how stressful my day is, so I don't have time.'

'I hate people who ask me to do something I didn't expect as it throws off my whole week.'

'Don't make me do that. I'd hate it afterwards even though at the time, I would love it.'

'I haven't got the time or the money.'

'I don't know how to.'

I will be honest with you here, I was so saddened by these replies. The act of being a little impromptu, which can result in so much fun, seemed so large and huge and immoveable to them. Maybe you will see yourself in one of these remarks – and maybe it will make you feel a little sad too.

For many people, it seems that routines begin to develop from packed-out schedules, and breaking from these schedules can be a very difficult thing; of course, we need to be at school, at work, on the bus, or on a train on time. Most of us, including me, have a calendar or a diary that we check and pop 'must-dos' into, but I'm here to tell you that those things in the calendar are things that we have to do. They're not the only things that we should do, though. If I get a last-minute call to do something and I have the time, I will jump on that opportunity, and I have had some of the best, most joy-inducing experiences this way. So we must seize the day more often and try to do something different.

I know that many of you reading this will immediately think I don't understand how busy your days are. But impromptu actions honestly can be possible and don't need to cost a penny either, as there are so many ways to be spontaneous that are free.

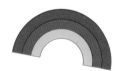

There *really* is nothing simpler to make you *happy* than doing something unexpected.

First, I want you to take a look at your diary and decide whether the things in there are essential, or if they're just in there because they're part of your usual routine. This might be difficult for you to do, but I want you to review it as objectively as possible and cross out anything that isn't necessary today. If you'd planned to go to a supermarket tonight because you always shop on Tuesdays, but you still have food in the fridge and could shop another day of the week, cross out that shopping trip. If you're due to go to a book club because you go every month, but you haven't read any of the books in six months and don't like half of the people that you attend with, don't go. You get the picture.

Now that you have cleared some time, use it to do something unexpected. Go for a walk somewhere that you haven't been before, visit that pub you've always wanted to go to, see that friend you haven't seen in months, or buy those theatre tickets that you've been wanting to get for weeks. The more 'out-there', the better!

If everything is essential, though, and your day is completely blocked out, why not find a few minutes (and I really mean just a few) to change what you usually do? The simple task of having something different for lunch could make the day less predictable and unsurprisingly special. I made a friend of mine, who's in a very stressful job that he hates, change up his daily food and he said that the easy task of not going to the same sandwich shop and buying the same wrap had made his day. In doing something unexpected, he felt like a rebel, which really made him smile. The smallest things can make a massive difference, so please do slot something in.

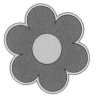

This principle can also apply with venues – if you're due to meet someone in a pre-planned location where you usually meet, why not change it up? I was going to meet up with one of my dearest friends who I hadn't seen for a couple of years due to the pandemic and we had our lunch all planned, which unsurprisingly included a walk, a talk and a meal. For various reasons, including the British weather, the plan changed at the last minute, so we instead met at the Victoria and Albert Museum. I have to be a bit museum-ist here and admit that my favourite museum is the V&A, so the idea of an excuse to wander around its great halls filled my heart with joy. My friend, however, likes to know everything that she's doing in advance and so was quite taken aback by the change in venue. When we met, she said she hadn't done anything like this for years, so I set her some Tiny Tasks, which you'll find below, and which she loved. I asked her whether she felt joy, to which she replied she'd always imagined joy to be about beaming smiles and shouting yay at every opportunity, and that while her feelings weren't like that, she certainly did feel happier. And if you break free from your routine, you will as well.

I urge you to please give one of these Tiny Tasks a go. Try the smaller things, and start to feel more joyful about your day.

Today's Tiny Tasks

These might feel tough for many of you, but please remember there are no rules here and I am not going to tell you off or frown if you can't do them all. All I ask is you give them a proper try.

1

Do the daring thing of changing what you eat for lunch today. If you make your lunch or buy it, please try something different. It doesn't mean spending a lot of money or eating something you've never had, all I mean is change that taste sensation. Why? It sparks joy! Obviously, it should be something you actually like to eat, otherwise where's the joy in that change?

2

Change your route to work, or school, or to the supermarket, on one day. Do it. Add 10 minutes onto your trip and go a different way. It's the simplest way to get somewhere you haven't been in a while, or possibly have never been. And even if you have been there before, you'll see new things along the way!

3

Phone a friend and ask them to meet in a totally different place to usual. I know that's a huge leap on from the above two Taskettes, but please try it. It doesn't have to be jumping on a train or plane (although if you have the money and the time, do that!). By changing it up with someone else you're spreading the joy, and that's what this is all about.

We all *need* to use the word 'NO' a *little* more.

The importance of *saying* 'no'!

There is another important thing that we all must try harder to do as we get older, and that is to use one of the most powerful words that you have available to you: NO! Toddlers seem to find this word very easy to say, but somewhere along the way, we lose the ability to use it.

Often we don't have the confidence to say 'no' to someone because we don't want to let them down, because we think others might not like us if we say it, or because we're worried that it might mean that we won't be not invited to do similar things again in the future. But saying 'yes' all the time is exhausting – it can lead to stress and burnout and certainly won't leave you with feelings of joy.

I'm here to give you a little nudge, to remind you that you can say no to something you don't want to go to. You can say no to a job you don't want. You are totally within your rights to tell friends that you can't be there tonight because you don't fancy it.

Saying no is something we all have to learn how to do again, and believe me when I say that I know that this is tricky to do – I like to say yes to people, in fact to everyone, but I am learning to say NO. Please believe me when I say that knowing you don't HAVE to do something that you really don't WANT to do is so empowering. We all need to use the word 'no' a little more.

Using your imagination

I have always had a very vivid imagination. When I was small, I imagined that I was on telly. In my head, I was hosting the children's TV show *Blue Peter*, or I was making people laugh. I would pretend all day. If I was ever called up to the front of the classroom, I would picture the other kids as my audience and imagine that I was on telly presenting whatever the teacher had asked me to talk about. It hugely helped with my shyness. I would go to sleep at night thinking about being on TV.

As the years went on, I would often sit at a table whilst 'revising' for my exams, looking out of the window for hours on end, imagining presenting many TV shows and hosting award ceremonies. And this brought me immeasurable joy.

I've been giving lots of advice around 'doing' things in this book, but here I would like to talk about the importance of our imagination. This is because our minds are immensely powerful. If we use our brains correctly, we can experience the joy that we get from actually doing something, purely by thinking about it and feeling it in our mind. So I really want you to start using it as much as you can.

We can experience
the joy that we get
from actually

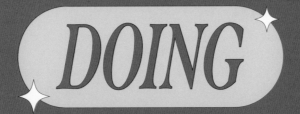

DOING

something,
purely by

THINKING

about it and feeling
it in our mind.

The problem is, though, our imagination is something that seems to disappear as an adult; I'm really not sure where it goes. Our imaginations are needed beyond the point that we are children and can help us do really exciting things! Whether it's taking part in the next series of *Strictly Come Dancing* or climbing up the Eiffel Tower, our imaginations can help us do them, in our heads. You have the ability to climb, fly, perform or become anyone you'd like to be. These imaginings are free and entirely our own: no one else can tell us what we can or can't dream up. And the most brilliant thing? As well as the immediate dopamine hit you get from doing something you've always wanted to in your mind, thinking about something so intently can often help you to set your sights on doing it in real life, too, and getting an even bigger joyful hit. It's a double whammy.

If you are unable to let your mind run riot, I do know a brilliant way to begin to engage it again. And that's through reading.

Every time I read a book I am the person within it, and I'm sure that this is the same for many people. When you read, you can become someone else, so it's a brilliant place to begin to flex your imagination muscles again. We do this through books when we are children, and we can still do it as adults.

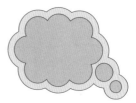

→ The magic of reading

I am extremely lucky that my parents and grandparents all loved books; I have been surrounded by them for my entire life. Everywhere you looked in my house, or that of my grandparents, was covered in books. I have vivid memories of reading as a very young child, both with my parents in the evenings before bed, and also on my own as I grew up. I loved and still love getting lost in a new world when I open my books. They helped me explore exciting new places and disappear from reality for a bit. As a child, I wanted to be Wendy in *Peter Pan*, or Alice, falling down that rabbit hole. I devoured best-selling new novels as a teenager, then when my mum suggested I read a classic, such as *Rebecca* by Daphne du Maurier and Emily Brontë's *Wuthering Heights*, I began, albeit slightly begrudgingly, to read them and, guess what, she was right, I fell in love with them too.

Reading is magical. It is so unlike any other media that we consume, because when we do it, we're not given any images. I genuinely love TV and films, but they put pictures right there in front of us and that doesn't fire our imaginations in the same way. A book makes you paint those pictures for yourself.

I understand that I come from a very privileged position here; many people think of reading as a chore, and I truly believe that's because reading is used in schools as a lesson, a method of teaching us to read and write, which is boring. The books that you may have had to read will not all have been fun, either. But, much like music, there are all sorts of genres of books out there, so why not visit your local library and borrow something new and unexpected? Libraries are places of wonder and of peace, and they give us the space to let our imaginations run wild again. They are free and hand us a place to be inspired – in my opinion, they're one of the most joyful places around.

Once you've got a book that you're interested in reading, the next challenge is to try to make time to read it (I know I find that difficult). Perhaps you could find a few minutes on your commute, before you go to bed, in your lunch break, or straight after you wake up? Find those few minutes each day to read another chapter or another ten pages. While you're reading, really build a picture of the characters and places in your mind. If the book doesn't describe how a place looks for you, that's okay – you can make it up for yourself (and, of course, while we are building our imaginations here, I would urge you to speak to your friends about good books that you've read, or to pass on or recommend a good book to someone else so that you can experience the joy of it together).

Now, how about we give our imaginations a spin, for old time's sake?

Why not start by opening your mind and revisiting something within it that you enjoyed as a child? No one is going to judge you. You're not going to be marked on how good the pictures that you draw in your mind are, so go as wild as you like. These thoughts are yours and yours alone – no one can take that from you. Once you've got the hang of it, it's there for you whenever you need it. I can guarantee you will be able to feel the joy, even if the act is entirely in your mind.

Today's Tiny Tasks

This Task is one to keep just for yourself. It's imagination time. Do these whenever or wherever you want. On the tube, bus, train, in bed, in the kitchen, walking, out with friends – in fact ANYWHERE, because this is one for you and you alone.

1

Imagine you are laughing. Yes, that's all. I want you to picture yourself having a giggle.

2

Next imagine that you're having a laugh, but now open your imagination and look at what you're laughing at. Don't just see it, really soak it up. Watch that scene for as long as you like. Stay in that imaginary world for a while and keep laughing.

3

Now I would love you to venture back in time and try to remember what you would imagine when you were small. Not those scary things or stuff that worried you as a child, this time it's winning the FA Cup, going on the world's biggest rollercoaster, hosting that TV show, being in the next Harry Potter movie, or whatever else comes to mind. Please try to go there in your head. Use that image that you have inside and welcome it back into your life.

Here's the little extra note that you don't have to do, but if you'd like to, give it a go. Write down or draw what you saw and the pictures you painted in your mind. Again, no one is judging you and there is no right or wrong way of doing this. This is just for you. If you would like to share it with a friend or a family member, do it. If you just want to tell them that opening up their imagination again will make them feel good, then you've just spread the joy!

● Abandon *your* social anxiety

Whenever I have to go to a party or an event, my shy fifteen-year-old self ends up materialising. House parties bring out the worst reaction in me, swiftly followed by any event that I'm not working at – oddly, if I don't have the distraction of work, then I'm not in 'work mode' and I get worried that I won't know what to say. As someone who never ever stops talking, I know that probably seems bizarre, but there we go – it's that fear of being judged or disliked all over again.

My fear was so extreme in the past that I have been known to get an upset stomach on the day before heading out. If I don't know anyone there, I can often be found grabbing my husband's hand very tightly. If he needs to go to the loo, he has found me following him. I hate to be left alone at these things. I know that this probably sounds insane to you; I can stand up on live TV (which I absolutely LOVE) or host a huge live event in a massive arena largely without fear, but I can't walk into a party. All I can say is that there are varying degrees of shyness, and for me, parties bring out my shy side. I'm sure that this resonates with many of you reading this.

I might get scared about going to parties, but when I get there and manage to come out of my shell, I often make new friends and have the best time. But how do I get to the parties when my fear is so crippling? I have learnt a few ways to cope over the years and I would love to share them with you – I am certain these will make you feel a little stronger in any social situation that you are feeling anxious about, be that a party, a visit to a pub or a networking event. Some of life's most joyful moments can be had with people, so don't lock yourself away because of your shyness.

First, unless you have a good reason to say no (see page 131 about saying NO if you truly don't want to go), say yes to the invitation. Don't think about it, just say yes. It will be worth it.

When the day rolls around, dress colourfully. I've provided some tips on page 36 about how to do this if you're a little nervous – but please do it, it will lift your spirits.

These are tips I have given many people and that have honestly worked!

From the moment you walk into that room/ pub/party, remember to smile. Walk in with a big grin on your face — not only is it a simple thing that will make you feel better, people may notice and think that you look lovely and friendly, which will help the next part!

Walk right up to someone who you don't know and say: 'Hi I am...'. If the person is also on their own, it's highly likely that they'll be relieved that you've spoken to them. So many times, people have replied to this with: 'Oh, thank goodness you said that as I know no one here.' Now you have a 'pal', someone that you can look around with and talk to.

I know you're probably thinking, 'But Gaby, now I'm stuck with this person who I don't know and I don't know what to say next!' People get really nervous about striking up conversation and learning more about someone, but there are a few simple questions you can ask to get the ball rolling. First, ask them what they do. Then tell them what you do. Ask questions about things that they've said, but don't forget to listen as listening is vital too. There you are, you are having a conversation.

Someone I recently gave this advice to said it had led to them meeting the dullest person in the room. I personally don't think anyone is dull or boring – you're just not asking them the right questions. Every single person has a story. If you ask them questions and listen to their answers – and I do mean really listen – you will learn something new and become more joyful in the process. You'll probably make the other person joyful too for giving them your attention. And, hey, if it still turns out that the person you're speaking to is very dull and boring, at least you've broken the ice.

If you don't want to start asking any questions without having a 'get out', here are some lines that may help:

'I'm so sorry, I need the bathroom, do excuse me.' (I know that's the oldest one, but it works!)

'You are so fascinating, but I feel like I have taken up too much of your time already, please excuse me I need to chat with...' (and point in the general direction of other people).

'Thank you so much, I can't tell you what a joy it's been to talk to you. It's thanks to you that I am now able to go and spread the joy.'

These tips can be life changing, believe me. I have a very old friend who is now married to the person they first spoke to at a New Year's Eve party that they were initially too nervous to go to. I said to them, 'You never know, you may meet the girl of your dreams.' And, yes, you guessed it, that is exactly what happened. So don't shy away from social situations – use these tips to manage your fear. Throw yourself in.

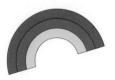

Chapter_

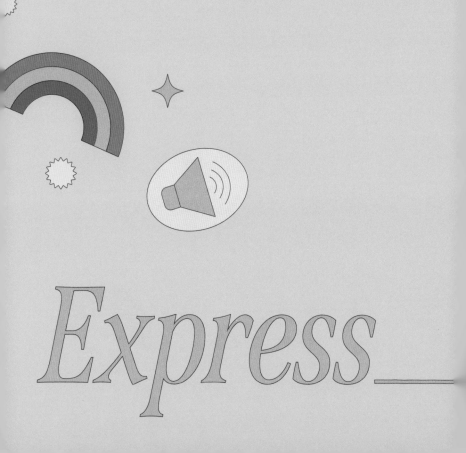

*Express_*

04

Yourself

So many people can't quite believe that I now shout from the rooftops about singing, jumping, dancing and skipping. As you've already read in this book, I was, and at times still am, very shy. Letting go, smiling and jumping around helps me and everyone I know to feel joy, but when I was younger, I was never the person who would go out of her way to do these things in public.

Dancing and singing are so powerful – they have helped me and my friends through some really difficult times. My lovely friend was recently diagnosed with breast cancer (it was caught very early, she's only young and she is doing so well) and she asked if I would come and sit with her during her chemo as she knew I would attempt to sing and dance around, which would make her feel better. Dancing is something that my late friend Deborah James kept doing throughout all of her treatments – even when she felt absolutely dreadful – and it made her, her family and all of her followers on social media feel more hopeful. Other friends have said that keeping smiling, dancing and mucking around have helped them cope with their treatments too. Expressing yourself in these ways can inject even the saddest of situations with more joy.

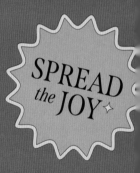

SPREAD
the JOY

BEING SILLY

and putting yourself out there
can be scary, but please do try
to abandon your fear here.

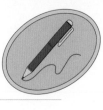

But here's the thing — we don't need to have a horrific diagnosis to be able to reap the rewards that dancing and singing can bring. Using them in our everyday lives can be a brilliant way to make us all feel joy more often.

Of course, it's not possible for us to dance, sing and skip 24/7 – that would annoy everyone, and that's where the rest of the chapters in this book come in – but while we are able to, we should express ourselves as much as possible. If you like nothing better than singing along to Britney Spears whilst finishing a jigsaw, then blooming well do it. You may be wondering why I randomly mentioned Britney at that moment? Well, a song of hers just came on the radio and I found myself singing along loudly to it and my husband called from the other room wondering what I was doing. I said, 'My book and singing Britney, why?' He laughed!

So, this chapter is about letting go and expressing yourself. Now that I've said that, I realise that some people might want to run away. Being silly and putting yourself out there can be scary, but please do try to abandon your fear here. Just head straight in and remember, I have your back (metaphorically, of course).

● Music

Music is very important to me, and I know many people feel the same way. I'm confident that music in some form – whether it's:

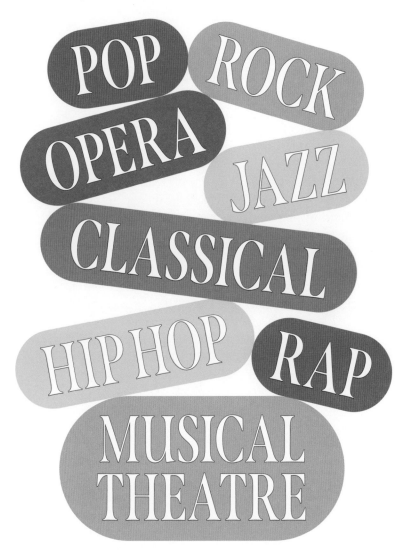

POP ROCK OPERA JAZZ CLASSICAL HIP HOP RAP MUSICAL THEATRE

or perhaps even just a beat – will have accompanied you throughout some of your most formative moments.

On a personal level, music has been central to my joy throughout my life. From singing along to musicals in my bedroom as a child, to the records that I now play on the radio, I have always loved nothing more than putting on my favourite songs whenever I need a little burst of happiness; in fact, I am currently listening to the soundtrack of *A Chorus Line* (if you were wondering) as I write this, to keep me feeling jolly as I work. My family are similar to me in this regard; we often use music to feel more joy in our days. Every morning, my husband plays his favourite songs when he's in the shower to set himself up for the day, and my dad always used to listen to opera (rather than musicals, like me) in the early evenings when he was working. I am not an opera fan by any stretch of the imagination, but I liked hearing it when it came on, as I knew it brought him joy.

While there are certain genres of music I like more than others, the pieces that mean the most to me are the ones that bring the memories of moments from my past, and all the emotions that I felt during them, to the surface. I remember going on a date with a guy who I really fancied, who played 'The Whole of the Moon' by The Waterboys in the car. That song gives me goosebumps to this day. (By the way, we only ended up dating for about six weeks – he wasn't really what I hoped he'd be and neither was I what he was hoping for – but this is the power of music!) Going even further back in time, I fancied all of the members of The Police and had posters of them all on my walls, so whenever I hear a song by them, I blush! And so many songs I hear nowadays from the 90s and noughties take me back to the TV shows I was hosting at that time and the guests that came on them – every Take That song makes me smile because they were always on the Saturday morning kids' show *Motormouth* that I presented. It's a really special experience to listen to all of these.

Unlock a happy memory

Even if you don't love listening to music in your leisure time, I'm certain that some pieces of music will make you feel very powerful emotions when you encounter them. Music has a very strong connection with memory; you may notice this when you find yourself crying after hearing a song that was played at a loved one's funeral, even if it was years and years ago, or when you feel warmth radiate from your heart when you hear the song that accompanied your first date. Songs can remind us of moments in our past, or of hidden memories that lurk deep within our subconscious – and when we unlock these memories, they can bring immense joy.

So I would really like you, right now, to get up and put some music on that you enjoy, or that you know will unlock a happy memory. It could be a song that you treasure from earlier on in your life, or it could simply be something that you enjoy listening to. I'd like you to just sit and listen to it until it's over and do nothing else at all while you're doing so – it doesn't need to be very long. Perhaps close your eyes and let the song, and the emotion you feel from it, really wash over you. If you can't think of anything at all, why not listen to one of my favourite joy-inducing songs?

'Angelina'
Louis Prima

'I Feel Good'
James Brown

'Reach'
S Club 7

'Happy'
Pharrell

'Don't Stop Me Now'
Queen

'All About You'
McFly

'It's Not Unusual'
Tom Jones

'Let Me Entertain You'
Robbie Williams

'You Can't Stop the Beat'
Hairspray movie cast

'Livin' la Vida Loca'
Ricky Martin

'Surfin' USA'
Beach Boys

'Feel It Still'
Portugal. The Man

'You're the First, the Last, My Everything'
Barry White

'Uptown Funk'
Mark Ronson/
Bruno Mars

By listening to this music, you have not just engaged in a short-term *joy-boosting* activity; the benefits of music go far beyond the personal. Indeed, the multitude of effects that music can have on our brains are still being studied, and can be *very powerful*.

→ *The positive power of music*

I play music at every opportunity during the day. First thing in the morning, I'll turn on the radio and listen to a breakfast radio show – I'll often choose Radio 2 with Zoe Ball, or Virgin with my old TV partner in crime Chris Evans, because they play my type of music and engage in my kind of chat and laughter. When I work out, I play music. When I am in the car, I play music. While I typed this, I was playing music (a medley of Broadway shows over the years is a very popular choice). Music is already known to reduce stress, pain and symptoms of depression, to boost our immune systems and help repair brain damage, and also to improve our cognitive and motor skills. It is even beginning to be understood to have a profoundly positive effect on patients with Alzheimer's and Parkinson's disease, where research has shown that emotionally significant pieces of music can help people recall memories. I have never forgotten how incredible it was to see a beautiful, frail elderly woman brought back to her old smiling self when a music specialist played his guitar for her and she slowly lifted her head, smiled and started to sing. Together they sang her favourite song from when she was a young girl. She remembered nothing else and most of the time she couldn't even speak, but when he played his guitar she was that young girl again and she was free.

Music really is so magical, and the best thing about it is that there is no 'right' music to listen to in order to achieve its health benefits; you don't need to only listen to classical music to improve your cognitive skills (like we used to believe) – studies have recently shown that any music you enjoy can unlock them.

I promise that listening to more of the

MUSIC YOU LOVE

every day will make you feel more JOYFUL.

Taking the time to listen to the music is incredibly good for you.

The next time that you're feeling a little low, why not reach for one of those songs that you know will lift your spirits?

When you're doing something that you don't really enjoy, why not put on a tune that might make it more fun?

And the next time you begin your day, why not listen to a song that you love, just like my husband does, so that you can start it out right? I promise that listening to some more of the music you love every day will make you feel more joyful.

Now, I know that some of you might now be thinking: 'But what if the music that I want to listen to isn't the music that others enjoy?' If you aren't able to listen to your music on your own through headphones, then, simply, I would like you not to pay attention when someone makes a comment about what you're listening to – there is no such thing as good or bad music. That's it. If you must reply, you could say, 'It's good for my brain and this is the music I love, so it's doing me good AND it's putting a smile on my face.' They might even learn to appreciate your music, which could enable them to feel joy too, or they might simply be able to feel happy that you are feeling joy from it. Either way, keep listening to what you love, and make time for it whenever you can.

Sing

I have always loved singing. When I was little, I was always in my room using my hairbrush as a microphone. I wasn't pretending to be a pop star, oh no. For me it was musical theatre all the way. I would learn every single part and then sing it at the top of my lungs. This brought me huge joy, even if it brought my parents huge earache. When people at school said which bands they loved, I would always join in, but as well as reeling off my favourite bands from *Top of the Pops*, I would talk about my favourite musicals. (My daughters both love musical theatre, too, and I can't work out why…!) Some kids at school got me and some just thought that I was odd, but I didn't care. Singing along to shows has honestly always brought me joy. I was lucky enough to be in the stage show *Chicago* as Mama Morton for a while in London's West End, and as you can imagine it was unbelievably exciting for me to be there singing on that stage!

> Today, I sing everywhere and anywhere I can with no shame.

I have even been known to see a street sign and burst into song: there's a street I walk by called Chitty Street, and each time I see it I can't help myself but start singing 'Oh, you, pretty Chitty Bang Bang'. Some people would probably rather crawl into a corner and hide than do this, but not once has anyone ever said anything horrible to me about my singing in the streets. Many times complete strangers join in with me, and the joy I feel when someone suddenly sings along is amazing.

Today,
I sing

everywhere
& anywhere

I can with
no shame.

→ *Group dynamics*

Over time I have realised that singing is not just something that I love to do, it is one of the most joy-enhancing things that anyone can easily do at any point of the day. Like music, singing relieves stress, which, of course, helps you feel more relaxed. And that in turn helps you cope with everyday situations in a calmer and better way. Like exercise, it makes the brain release the feel-good hormone oxytocin, which helps to reduce anxiety. And what's even better is that singing in a group has been found to bring people together – you can literally strengthen your sense of connection with strangers just by belting out a tune. My husband, who is a football fan, always talks about the joy he feels when at a match the fans sing together, and everyone starts smiling. So by singing, you'll feel more joyful, which helps you to help others feel more joy.

→ *You have permission to sing*

I know there's a certain amount of embarrassment that people feel when I tell them to try singing. Everyone is worried they'll be judged – that someone will put their fingers in their ears and tell them to stop. So many people think they can't sing. But guess what? You can! It doesn't matter whether you are young or old, whether you have a high or a low voice, or if you can hit notes pitch perfect – you can open your mouth and make a sound. And by singing, you can feel joy. So, regardless of whether you think of yourself as a singer or not, I am giving you the permission to sing. Do it! Try it. You will feel better.

First, I want you to try to take away your fear of singing. It gets in the way of so much. Imagine right now that you're not scared to sing. How do I do this? Well, I think that any piece of music was written just for me to perform. I pretend that no one is there or listening – sometimes I close my eyes to help with that – and then I open my mouth and let it out. Try it for yourself. I promise, the joy you will feel is truly magical.

A final, fun added benefit of singing is that it helps with snoring. Now snoring can be a bit of a joy sapper, especially if your partner happens to do it and keeps you up all night… so imagine the joy that singing could bring if it not only made you happier in the day, but also at night! Yep, that kinda joy makes me smile hugely. In short, we should all sing more.

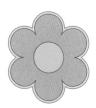

Singing in public

Something really rather special happened when I was travelling on the tube recently.

I was standing up midway through the train and a young man was listening to some music through his headphones and humming loudly. For some reason, there seems to be an unwritten rule about making a noise on public transport, where people often think that they'll bother others if they do it. But no one minded, and I watched as more and more people looked up and smiled. When he looked up, he saw us all smiling and started singing the words out loud. It was unmistakably Bon Jovi's hit 'Livin' on a Prayer'. Slowly, I joined in with him and then others joined in too and he then stood up and we all started singing together. We all sang at the top of our lungs, and when it was over we cheered and clapped and smiled at each other. This wasn't a pre-arranged flash mob, it was one man and his voice bringing everyone together and spreading joy. Everyone was smiling afterwards. So the next time you're listening to some music that means a lot to you, why not share it with others by singing it out loud?

Today's Tiny Tasks

Do not cringe or shudder at these Tasks. Yes, it's SINGING (but not like you've ever sung before!). Choose your favourite song and try these. Each of the three ideas should be taken and tried over three consecutive days.

1

Sing out loud. Sing that song in the privacy of your bedroom. I'm not talking about whisper-singing when I say sing, I mean belt it out. Spread your arms and sing from the heart. No one is watching, no one can hear you. Just do it.

2

Stand on the street and hum that same song just gently out loud. Don't look around at anyone, look at the sky or the view, but hum out loud.

3

You may have guessed what comes next, but please just try. Sing just a few words out loud when you're out and about. Once you've done this it will make you smile. If other people are around, they might smile back. Who knows, when you get used to singing on the street, someone might just join in. Imagine the joy you would have spread with that one simple moment!

Throw caution
to the wind

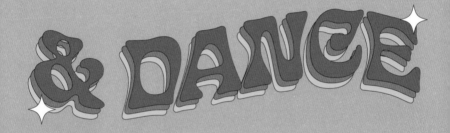

at every
opportunity.

● Dance

For so many years I was self-conscious about absolutely everything: my short and big arms; my freckles; my height (I've been 5 foot 8 and three-quarters since I was twelve – quite tall at a young age!). But I was particularly self-conscious about dancing – not only was I not confident in my body, I was shy, and, worst of all (in my mind) I couldn't remember any dance steps, which made me horribly embarrassed. I hated the idea of letting go and dancing all night long. For years, I'd heard my dad telling people that he couldn't dance, so before long I found myself telling people the same thing in order to avoid the embarrassment of dancing in public, but I was able to move in time with the music, so that wasn't true. (In actual fact, only a tiny percentage of the global population are genuinely unable to move in time with a beat, so if you've been using this excuse to stop dancing too, please know that it's highly unlikely that you genuinely can't dance, and it's actually your fear that is getting in the way here, like mine was with me.)

I went to drama college after A levels, which I loved, and where we had to do dance classes in front of a mirror at the start of every day, which did awful things for my self-consciousness. Yes, I stood right at the back and tried to hide the fact that I just couldn't remember to go left, left and turn (you get the picture).

At Guildford (the drama school I attended) we had a weekly class called 'Presentation', where we would perform a solo song that we'd worked on to our tutor and our classmates. I loved this hour, as it meant that I could sing musical theatre songs, but one week I chose 'The Music and the Mirror' from *A Chorus Line*, one of my favourite musicals (which, in fact, I am listening to right at this moment – oh how I love this show). The song is about being a dancer and showing others your dancing skills. Yes, considering my fear of dancing I can see the irony in choosing the song, but I was desperate to perform it. When I told my teacher that was what I planned to present, they quite rightly said that I should move while singing. By 'move' she didn't mean dance, but I knew that this was a number that a dancer sings, and in my head I wasn't a dancer. So, in the end, I chose not to present it.

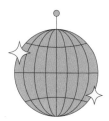

I know it seems silly to say this now, so many years later, but I have always loved that song, and I wish I hadn't been so self-conscious of my dancing that it prevented me from singing it on that stage. I know now that no one would have been judging me for my dancing; they would likely have all been too worried about how they looked for their own presentations and ignored me entirely.

But a good thing did come out of this story. My history of self-conscious dancing has made me want to throw caution to the wind and dance at every opportunity. I might not be able to follow steps, but I can move. I was often prancing around in the streets, and thought it would be funny to film videos of me doing this. Off the back of this, something very strange and thrilling has begun to happen to me. I now have complete strangers coming up to me in the streets and asking if they can dance with me. If you don't follow my Instagram account (and why should you?) I have posted many videos in which I'm acting the fool and jumping around to music. I don't think that what I'm doing is even vaguely dancing, but I'm going to use that term lightly anyway.

One lovely woman recently started chatting to me while she was out shopping with her daughter. She told me that she had always wanted to just dance around in the street but had never had the courage to do so. She had followed me on Insta and had hoped to bump into me so that we could dance together – so we did. She chose the song, and outside St Paul's Cathedral in the City of London she and I jumped around. Her daughter filmed us and at the end she said, 'Mum, I am so proud of you.' There's a moral to this tale: life's too short not to jump around. What's stopping you? If you can let go and smile you will spread joy AND feel proud of yourself, so why not jump and dance? It is liberating.

I now dance with all sorts of lovely people in the streets, but I still would never and will never do *Strictly*. I don't want to dance around with someone scoring me and voting. I'm not about anyone judging me for my dancing – I dance because it's all about fun and joy.

So, I'd love you to release your inner child – the next time you feel you need a little boost, or just that you want to show people how happy you are, please jump, skip or leap around to some music (whether you're playing it out loud or if it's in your head). In doing so, you'll be dancing and spreading the joy too.

WHAT'S STOPPING YOU?

If you can let go and smile you will spread joy AND feel proud of yourself, so why not jump and dance?

It's liberating.

Today's Tiny Tasks

Put on a song you can move to. Please don't think too long about it – as with your other Tasks, just take the embarrassment out of this one. Notice I am not using the word 'dance' here, as people fear that word, thinking that they need to be as good at it as the professionals on *Strictly Come Dancing*. So choose a joyful dance-along song and move and jump around to it. Dancing will make you feel more energised, and you will go into your next part of the day with your blood pumping around a little faster. You probably won't be able to stop that smile, knowing that you've just danced like no one was watching, and you will start to pass on that joyful energy.

1

Move gently to some music that you pop on.

2

Dance and throw your arms around and smile, but do this on your own in the privacy of your home or in a quiet place at work.

3

Ask someone to join you. Try this at work – you'll be amazed at the number of people who'll give you one of 'those' looks but then will eventually join you. Or simply ask a friend round and when they get there just say, 'Fancy a dance?', then put the music on and move around the room.

PS If you're feeling confident, maybe try dancing and leaping around in the street? Go on, you know you want to!

Take up something *new*

One of my favourite subjects at school was art. I would doodle anywhere, anytime. I loved to draw and I really loved pottery. As you may gather, it's been quite a while since I did my exams… I was fifteen when I took them (my birthday is in July, so I was one of the youngest in my year), at which point I passed pottery and never really made another pot or picked up a paintbrush for many, many years.

My next encounter with art happened about fifteen years ago when one of my lovely friends had a heart attack (he's fine, I hasten to add). I went to see him in hospital and, feeling inspired by my childhood love, I took him an easel, some paints and a sketchbook. I told him to stop partying and paint. He laughed, we laughed together, and I don't think he listened to me. I didn't even listen to myself! So I quickly forgot all about art again.

Then, about eight years ago, I was taking my elder daughter to an art shop for her GCSE exams when I was suddenly taken back to being at school. I instantly remembered how much I used to love pens and paper and paints. We left that day with not only the stuff my daughter needed, but also with a sketchbook for me and some watercolour pens. I was so excited to give art a go again.

I came home and hung the bag on the back of a door, waiting till the weekend to get everything out. When Saturday rolled around, I grabbed the pens and started work in that pad. I felt so liberated about the fact that I wasn't being judged; all I was doing was making myself happy. The first thing I drew was a jar of mayo. The next was a flower, and then a chair. Not very exciting things, I'll admit, but they were very simple and I loved it.

I have carried on doodling, drawing and having fun with pens and art ever since. My husband even proudly got one of my quick watercolour pen drawings framed recently; it's of a parakeet, and I must admit I am rather proud of it. The joy it brought my husband was certainly palpable – he'd never known the side of me that doodled. I felt thrilled and delighted that he liked it.

The power of new

In taking up art again, I have realised that getting yourself a new hobby, or even taking up something from our past, can be such a lovely joyous thing. It doesn't have to cost you anything to get started, and if you have decided to do something creative, you don't have to show anyone what you make. Perhaps, like me, you'd like to give drawing a go? Or maybe it's knitting, cross stitch, card making, writing, colouring, or even playing an instrument? The important thing is that whatever you choose should make you smile. Set aside a time to do it when you want to relax – I'm certain it will help.

We're too quick to abandon hobbies in our adulthood; I bought a set of pens for my friend the other day as she was having a tricky time, and I thought they might lift her spirits. They did and she showed me her doodles. She said she hadn't used felt tips for years and asked me why I hadn't told her that these pens were going to bring her so much joy. That's why I've added this to the book. I'm sharing my joy and hers, and in the process passing it on to you.

Confidence, I realise, is something that we need much more of as we get older. We need to be given permission to do those things that brought us simple joy as a child. So it might feel as though I'm stating the obvious, but here I am, giving you that permission! If you're happy with what you create, why not show it to someone else, or give it to them as a gift? Or perhaps, like me, you could even gift some pencils or pens the next time that someone is feeling sad? That way, you can keep passing on the joy.

MY SCHOOL REPORTS *ALWAYS* USED TO SAY THE SAME TWO THINGS.

GABY
DOESN'T
STOP
TALKING
AND ALL
SHE DOES
IN CLASS
IS *GIGGLE*.

Laugh

Laughter is truly the best medicine; I'm sure that I don't need to tell you that. I believe that the best type of laughter is the one that flows from you uncontrollably – perhaps when a friend tells you a funny story, when you're watching a comedy, or when you simply get the giggles and you can't stop, so much so that when you try to stop all you do is laugh more, leaving you literally exploding with laughter, crying and unable to breathe. I have always been a huge giggler. My school reports always used to say the same two things. Gaby doesn't stop talking and all she does in class is giggle. I have often found myself in situations where I wished the ground would open up and swallow me because I really, truly cannot stop laughing. And when someone gives me one of those stern looks asking me to be quiet – that makes me giggle even more. Afterwards, though, I always feel brilliant about having let my happy emotions show.

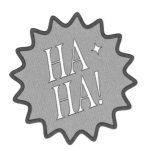

→ *Don't fake it*

Like fake joy, fake laughter is a big NO-NO – it won't make you happy, or anyone around you. In this section, I won't be telling you to laugh more – doing so would only make you agonise over finding things funny, which won't help anyone. Instead, I'm going to include just one simple tip, which is to put yourself in front of the things that you know will get you laughing whenever you need a little burst of joy. Give yourself permission to stop and have a giggle. Social media these days can be awash with funny short videos and bloopers, and they really can make you feel better. So if you're scrolling, don't scroll past them; watch them, and if you love them, share that laughter by sharing it with your family and friends, too.

Three memories that always make me laugh

I'm going to share three stories from my personal life that really make me laugh, in the hope that they might tickle you. Before I go any further, I need to mention that no one was actually hurt when taking part in the various things I am going to share here. Okay, on we go, and I need you to use your imagination and picture yourself there with me.

→ Oh yes, you will!

One very silly time, many years ago, I was in panto (oh how I love pantos, oh yes, I do! Happy memories of seeing them with the family when I was little) and was lucky enough to be playing Cinderella. In all honesty, it wasn't the perfect role for me — I always fancied being Dandini or Buttons, if the truth be told — but there I was as Cinders singing the theme song of an Australian soap opera called *Home and Away* with Prince Charming and Buttons. Yes, you did read that right, we sang the words of a song that opened a soap opera on TV. We'd sung it together over many shows, but on this one night a fly landed on Prince Charming's nose while the lovely girl playing this character was singing. The fly had spent a long time circling over her head before it decided to perch right on the tip of her nose, and I completely lost it. Prince Charming didn't budge or try to swat the fly, which made it even funnier. I was on stage, and yet I became utterly hysterical and started behaving like a dribbling wreck. The ludicrous situation of singing that silly theme song to someone who was remaining professional throughout made the situation even more crazy. From the second that the fly landed on her nose, not one word came out of my mouth. At the end of the song I walked off, still weeping with laughter, and had to apologise to the actress. She was lovely and kind and didn't mind and kept giggling herself at my silliness. I think the audience may have seen the fly, but it didn't matter as they also laughed and laughed at me, because there's something about someone else losing it on stage in panto that makes the laughing contagious. Oh yes, it does...

The effect of laughing and, more importantly, laughing along with and together with others is something so special and incredibly powerful, and it is one of the most obvious ways of spreading joy.

→ Sliding on ice

My eldest daughter will be left embarrassed when I share this (but I did ask her for permission, so here goes). When she was little (probably around five) I took her ice skating. She was keen to skate off on her own, so I found a penguin (I don't mean a real penguin, obviously – don't be so silly – this was one of those plastic ones that kids hold onto to make sure they don't fall over) and told her it would be fine for her to hold onto it while I helped guide her around. Before I knew what was happening, though, she had gripped onto the penguin and had gone slipping off uncontrollably. Her penguin wasn't keeping her balanced at all and wouldn't stop moving. Rather than help, before long I was sitting on the ice in hysterics while she kept calling out, 'Mummy, Mummy, help! The penguin isn't saving me.' She became a bit of a fabulous skater by accident that day, with her little legs running to stay upright, even if she did use her ice skates more as running shoes than skates. Even the thought of it now makes me weep with laughter. (I do need to point out again that my daughter didn't actually hurt herself in the making of this story!)

When I was filming for the Saturday morning kids' TV show called *Motormouth* that I co-hosted for three years, I was asked if I would like to take part in a dramatic re-enactment of an air-sea rescue. As I am a bit of an adrenaline junkie, I said yes.

I was taken out in a small speedboat wearing a wetsuit and a buoyancy aid (it was March and I was being dropped off into the English Channel, so the wetsuit was very much appreciated). It was a slightly foggy day, so they had to take me further out than they had originally anticipated, which I thought was incredibly cool, fun and exciting. Before dropping me off, the filming crew reminded me that I had my mic on, and told me that if I was worried, I could just shout into it and they'd come back out to get me. Then I was popped into the sea; they waved and said the helicopter that would rescue me wouldn't be long. I waved back and saw them disappearing back to shore.

Before long, though, the fog thickened, leaving me unable to see them or the shore, and I started to get scared when I realised that I was alone, just bobbing around in the English Channel. I knew a helicopter would be coming to get me eventually, but I didn't know how long they'd be. So I decided I would start to sing (yep, back to singing!) to keep myself feeling okay. I apologised in advance to the camera crew, who could still hear me through my mic, and started to sing everything I could from *West Side Story*. The singing seemed to work — in fact, I was so distracted I didn't even notice my mic disconnect from my wetsuit and begin to float away. When I realised, I scrambled to get it, but it had disappeared. I also need to point out that I didn't have any other radio contact with my TV crew or with anyone else for that matter. I didn't have a walkie-talkie or anyone talking to me in my ears! I was properly ALL ALONE in the English Channel.

By this point, I was beginning to panic, which got even worse when I heard a loud (very, very loud) sound, and turned to see a huge ferry coming towards me. I thought about how daft I looked, bobbing in the water, singing songs, and started to giggle. Uncontrollable panicky laughter kept coming out of me. I then spotted a man hanging from a helicopter flying towards me and when he grabbed me up out of the water, I kissed him, giggled some more and asked if we could do it again. He later said that he'd never rescued anyone laughing so much and singing songs. But you know what, laughing (and singing) made me feel better.

Even if these stories haven't made you chuckle as much as they do me, they've certainly shown me the power of hunting for funny memories when you feel like you need a boost of joy. Why not spread that joy by telling other people your funny stories, too?

→ *Write your funny and daft memories below!*

_____

_____

_____

_____

_____

_____

_____

_____

_____

_____

_____

_____

_____

_____

_____

_____

_____

_____

❋ Jump

I'm beginning this section with a command: JUMP. Yes, I do want you to do it now, if you can. Stand up, take a breath in and jump. It doesn't have to be very high.

> How did that feel? Now, this time I'd like you to put your arms up in the air and jump again.

Fun, eh? Now that you've done that, I'd like you to jump one last time (for now) with your arms in the air and with a smile on your face. Jump! Don't worry, you're not doing this on your own. I am jumping with you – I have literally just got up from my computer to jump.

From performing that very simple movement three times, I know that your blood is now flowing a lot faster through your body – you're probably feeling a little more buzzy. I also know that the smile that you had on your face for your final jump is probably still there.

Jumping is one of the most joyful things in the world. I have been known to do it on my own, in company, or even when walking, often with my arms in the air, whenever I need a little boost. It is such a simple way to feel happier, but when I tell people this, so many people doubt that it will work. They think that jumping is stupid and silly. Really, I know that their reaction comes from a place of fear. So often, people are worried that others will see them and think that they're strange, or different, or odd. But if you're happy, what does it matter what people think?

Sometimes we really
need to give ourselves
permission to

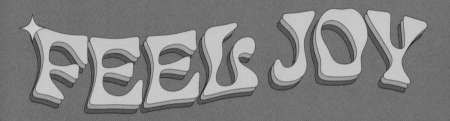

and make a conscious
decision to give
ourselves some joy.

→ Jump on your nervous feelings

One time, I was walking to a big TV meeting in town and was so nervous and desperate for the meeting to go well. I was doing what I usually do when I am nervous or worried: I pop a smile on my face, which often helps me feel better and in a lighter mood, and I employ the power of positive thinking by saying out loud to myself: 'You've got this, you can do it.' But I was still nervous. I suddenly realised I needed a jump, so I went for it. This might sound a little bizarre, but I have always jumped. When I was younger I used to jump just before doing a test at school or going to an audition. I think I must have read somewhere that it would help me; I honestly can't remember now. It's just something I have always instinctively done when I need a boost. But back to that jump on my way to a big meeting… I was in the middle of Hyde Park at the time (a very public place), and a very sweet couple asked me if I was okay, so I told them the truth: that I was a bit nervous about a meeting and I knew a jump would help. The lady laughed and said she thought I was mad, that jumping and smiling couldn't help me feel better about my meeting. Her husband, however, jumped with me. When she told him to stop, he did it again and so did I. She was so embarrassed. After a bit more jumping, though, we persuaded her to do it too. She laughed so much. We all did. That couple still contact me via Instagram and they now tell everyone they know that smiling and jumping helps. That's how simple it is to spread the joy.

Jumping clearly made an impact on this couple's lives, and yet because of how self-conscious they felt, they almost didn't do it! If we let fear get in the way of little things, how will we ever try bigger ones? Many people say that every day we should do something that scares us – these things really don't need to be big, a jump is all I am asking.

If I may, I would like to add in another jump story that happened only last week. I was walking through a park when I saw a young woman crying on a bench. I asked if she needed any help and sat down next to her; she told me her boyfriend had left her a couple of weeks ago and she thought she'd never feel happy again. We talked for a while, discussing all sorts before I asked her to stand up. I told her to trust me and that a simple jump would make her feel better. She really didn't want to, like many others, and told me it was silly. So I jumped without her. And as soon as I had, she got up and jumped herself. I told her to do it again, and we did, together. We kept jumping till we were both out of breath, and she laughed so much. She cried again afterwards as she said she'd thought that she'd never be able to laugh again, but now she realised she could.

Sometimes we really need to give ourselves permission to feel joy and make a conscious decision to give ourselves some joy. It really is allowed.

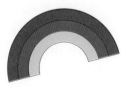

Today's Tiny Tasks

Before you leave your home, JUMP. Yes, it's that simple. Just jump. It doesn't matter how high or how silly you feel, do it, please.

Jumping releases those good feelings and I find it to be a particularly effective thing to do before leaving home. It will have you feeling better about your day from the minute that you leave. Many of us don't want to go to work, to school, to see the doctor, go to the supermarket, but putting that spring in your step automatically makes you feel that little bit brighter. And let's be honest, every single little thing we can do helps. You then leave home feeling better and you'll pass it on.

Here are your JUMP tasks. Please do these over a few days. Once you've mastered them, I'd recommend jumping whenever you feel that you need a little boost!

1

Jump inside your home. Do it in that moment before you open your front door. Then when you feel okay about this, jump after you've walked through the door, on your front doorstep. After you've upgraded to doorstep jumping, jump when you're outside.

2

Step outside, walk further than just where you live and jump with your arms in the air. Do it once, then the next time you try it maybe do it twice or a few times. But do it.

3

Finally, jump, smile and shout out YES! It might take a while for you to get over the fear of people looking at you, but you can do it. And trust me, it's worth it.

So, you guessed it, I would like you to jump, please, whenever you're feeling a bit miserable. And if you think you can't, ask yourself this – is that because you're worried about what people will think, or because you don't feel ready to let yourself feel joy yet?

Chapter_

Spread_

05

_the Joy

It might feel a bit strange to have an entire chapter dedicated to 'spreading the joy' – you're probably thinking that this is exactly what we've been talking about the whole way through this book. This, of course, is true. As you know by now, joy is infectious – while we have explored the fact that helping ourselves can make others happy, which in turn can make us feel even happier, we haven't yet spoken about how helping others directly can help us to feel more joyful. So I thought it would be important to dedicate this section to exactly that.

Now, I understand that we can live in a bit of an odd state of affairs sometimes; we worry that we will be judged if we don't help others, and at other times we worry that we'll be judged even more harshly if we help too much. (I'm sure we have all overheard those conversations where people go on about someone being annoyingly over-helpful!) And sometimes we can feel an immense amount of guilt purely because helping someone makes us feel happy. But it doesn't have to be this way. Just think – if we were all helping others, nobody would be able to judge anybody, and we wouldn't feel these levels of worry or guilt. There would be no one to point fingers at about helping too little or too much. Instead, nobody would be able to say anything other than thank you. If you get one thing from this part of the book, please take this: making time to give to other people will make the world more joyful in the long term, and in the short term it will make their day and yours too.

✳ Abandon the guilt

I've believed in helping people since I was a tiny girl; my mum taught me to be there for others and to always ask if they needed help. It's a rule that I've lived my life by ever since. It makes me feel joyful to know someone else feels better, or happier and warmer, or more cared for because of my actions. So I'm going to ask you to do the same here, because it will make them and you feel happier.

Being there for others can take many different forms. Indeed, one of the simplest and cheapest things that you can give to someone is your time. I will always try to have a chat with anyone I see who is looking a bit lonely, and I have a dear friend who rushes over to chat to anyone who is homeless. So many would just walk straight by, and not listen to the lives and stories that these people have to tell – and if you're able to buy them a cuppa, that's even better. And please, remember to ask their name, it really does mean the world to a homeless person. Many times they have said, when I ask their name, that it helps, because they feel invisible. It's a very simple thing to do. You will see them smile and in turn you feel good too.

Giving to others can mean offering up an ear or your expertise, or it could mean buying a coffee for someone or giving a donation – whether that's by going through your wardrobes and cupboards, or giving some money to a charity. Whatever you share will help others, and will make you feel good.

Some people hate to admit that you get a double-whammy of joy spreading when you give something to someone – they feel guilty that helping others makes themselves feel good. I'm not ashamed to admit that helping people makes me feel happy, and you shouldn't be either. Of course, helping others isn't a singularly selfish pursuit. If we encounter someone who needs our help, we shouldn't decide that we're just not going to help today because we're already feeling joyful enough, thank you very much, in a similar way to how we might decide to walk past a gym when we don't think that we need to exercise. There are many organisations, charities and people who are desperate for help, and I'd like to encourage you to give that help whenever you can. But I don't want you to feel guilty for helping when you do feel good about it. We all spend far too much time worrying that what we are doing is selfish, or that we will be judged. If giving to others makes you feel good, then that's okay! You're not being selfish and you are without a doubt spreading the joy.

I'm not going to suggest a Task to do here, because the best kind of help is whatever you choose to give. Instead, I would just love you to be more aware of the needs of others, and try to be the person who gives. When you give, consider how it makes you feel (without feeling guilty), and maybe even share the fact that helping has made you feel so much better with the person you are helping. Joy is a gift that you have – keep spreading it for all to see!

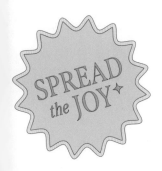

Friendship

Our busy, modern world can be an easy place to get lost in and feel as if you are on your own – but I truly believe that surrounding yourself with good friends is one of the most effective ways to be joyful. And I'm not alone; during the years of the Covid pandemic and lockdown, many people suddenly remembered how important friends are. Friends allowed us to break the monotony of our day-to-day existence; they were the first people that we joined Zoom calls with, and we tried our hardest to see them again whenever lockdowns lifted. I had certainly got into a habit of letting my friendships drift prior to the pandemic – perhaps you did too. Maybe you were left wondering why a friendship didn't feel the same any more? We spend many hours watching TV shows or movies that seemingly contain 'perfect' friendships – the type we all dream of, where people don't speak to each other for months on end but still have as good a time when they meet up again, where they can finish each other's sentences but still give each other the time and space to be their own person.

GOOD FRIENDSHIPS, like this, are some of the most **JOYFUL** things in the world, but behind the scenes, they take **WORK!** Now that we are in a post-pandemic world, it's **IMPORTANT** that we continue to give our friendships the **TIME** and **ATTENTION** that they deserve.

→ Be a good friend

What's the secret to being a good friend? It's a simple fact that in order to be a good friend both you and your friend need to be giving to the relationship. In my opinion, the two most important things that you can give in a friendship are a willingness to listen – no matter how big or small the thing is that they want you to listen to – and to help whenever you can. Doing both of these things, often, will result in trust and a real sense of connection growing within your relationship. I surely can't be alone in how much joy I feel when I can give my help and guidance to a friend. Of course, friendships can't be one-sided – you need to know that your friend is there to help you and is willing to listen, too. There's an expression that is so often banded about: 'I know I could call them at 3am and they'd come running.' If you have this, I am sure you've spent time nurturing that relationship. But there are many people who really aren't as lucky.

Perhaps you're one of these people who doesn't feel as though they have someone who has their back. If you are, I imagine you may be feeling rather lonely, and that's understandable, as the world is a huge place! Just the fact that you've been able to admit that you feel alone is progress; saying 'I feel lonely' is one of the most powerful statements you can make out loud and it takes such courage to admit that's how you feel.

My first piece of advice here is to be brave. Be the person who says hello. Maybe you can speak to someone that you like at work? Or maybe you can call a friend that you'd like to be closer to? I know that these things are difficult; it's much more tempting to scroll through Instagram 'liking' people's posts and hoping someone will 'like' yours back, but we all know that this sort of validation is a quick fix. Nothing beats a true, in-person relationship, so be the person who talks to others and asks for help. If you're feeling really lonely, there are places you can turn to. Don't forget there's a list of amazing charities at the back of this book that are there to help you.

If you are lucky enough not to feel alone, do you know someone who you suspect may be lonely? Is there someone in your life who has reached out to you, and who you just haven't found the time to speak to? Please find a few moments to call them – a 'Hello, how are you?' is all it takes. And you'll never know what new friends you'll make by doing this.

I had a meeting with someone only recently. She works in my industry and I have known her over the years but never spent time alone with her over a cup of coffee. We chatted and we talked and we laughed. When I got home, I said to my husband how much I liked her and realised I wanted to see her again as I thought we could be friends. A week later I saw her at an event when we bumped into each other. I took the bull by the horns and said how much I had loved spending time with her and she said she felt the same. We did gush a bit, and both admitted we had said to our husbands we thought we had found a new friend. We text now, and I feel blessed to have her in my life.

Here's the funny thing; when I told my husband about this, he told me that he thought women could be honest in this way but that men find it trickier. Men are taught that they're not able to be vulnerable, and so they feel more reluctant to look someone in the eye and say, 'I think I have a new friend,' or ask, 'Could we be friends?' I know this isn't a problem that just applies to men; we are all a little too worried that the other person might not feel the same. But if we spend less time worrying about what they think, and instead take time to be honest with ourselves and them, lovely friendships can happen. Wouldn't it be wonderful if you met someone who 'got' you, that you could then instantly tell just how much you enjoyed spending time with them?

I must, of course, point out that there will always be times when the other person doesn't feel the same, or where you don't want to meet up with someone again, but we learn from those too!

Good friends bring each other joy. Shared experiences are really special. So give your time to your friends and put work into those relationships.

Manners

My late mum was a stickler about good manners, and so is my dad. My mum said that the three simplest things to bring happiness to someone were the words 'please', 'thank you' and 'excuse me'. If we visited a country for our holidays, she always said we needed to learn those three phrases in their language. It's something I have passed on to my kids.

I was umming and ahhing about writing about manners. When I told some people that I wanted to include a section on this, a few said that they were an old-fashioned idea, but important. I truly think that manners bring joy, as they show that you are giving your respect to someone. And do you know what the funny thing is? When I asked those people who said that manners were old fashioned how they felt about someone not saying thank you, they told me that drives them mad. So, let's talk about manners – they are one of the simplest things that you can give to someone to make them feel appreciated, and therefore more joyful.

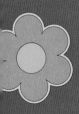

→ *Two very easy words*

'Thank you' can make such a massive difference in someone's day. My husband always tells me I say thank you too many times, but I don't think it's possible to say it too much. I want to show the other person that I appreciate what they have done for me. It doesn't matter how big or small the thing is that I'm thanking someone for – I even say it when someone steps aside to let me past on the street (if you live in a big city, you'll know that people prefer to just keep their heads down and not engage in conversation when they're walking); nine times out of ten they respond with a 'you're welcome' or just a smile. I know that by smiling and saying thank you for something that someone does, I am spreading joy. We all want to feel appreciated; saying thank you does just that.

Try it; if you've got into the habit of not saying thank you, please say it next time you go for your coffee. I spoke to a young girl in a high-street coffee shop, who was getting more and more frustrated as she made and handed out hot drinks, and not one person thanked her. With my interfering head on, I asked her if anyone ever said thank you. She told me that there are many days where no one says please or thank you at all. Days can go by when no one even looks at her. I found this really shocking and sad.

When did we become like this? Is it that we all just 'expect' too much? Or are we just too wrapped up in our own worlds? Take a moment to think, if this is you, what is your reason for not saying please or thank you? Psychologically, we all feel better when someone appreciates us, so let's make sure that we're appreciating others, too.

Today's Tiny Tasks

These may possibly be the most simple Tasks I ask you to try, but even so, they are ones you may find yourself not remembering to do.

1

When you get handed something, say thank you and look at the person as you say it.

2

When you ask for anything, say please, either at the end or the beginning of the sentence.

3

When you have to rush past someone, always say excuse me.

I know the above Tasks seem easy, and I can imagine you raising your eyebrows, but when you are tasked with doing them, you may just realise the number of times you don't!

Asking for help *and* helping others

This may seem like an odd one, but have you ever really thought about how often you ask for help? Or about the way you ask for help? You very well may wonder how you could possibly spread the joy simply by asking for help, but think about it, if you're trying to do everything yourself, you're really going to struggle to feel joyful. Has someone ever asked you to do something in a way that has made you feel angry, annoyed and not happy at all? I know people have asked me to do things in this way. So asking for help in the right way is important.

My late Granny (who I mentioned earlier in the book) was the most incredible woman who made a massive impact on everyone around her. Oh goodness me, I miss her so much. She used to gently push your hand away if you tried to help her. She was someone who looked after others and the idea that she needed a hand or any help drove her mad. I am aware I do the same; if someone asks if they can help (it happened the other day when my paper shopping bag split), I always say, 'No, I am fine,' but of course I need help. Especially when it comes to my computer (and anything maths-related, if I'm truthful) – so this section is for me, too!

Asking for a favour can feel like a huge thing. People keep their needs hidden for many reasons, with the most obvious being that they don't want to be perceived as weak or incapable. Why do we not want to look weak? I think it's built into us as women that we want to show we can be as strong as anyone; men, on the other hand, feel that they need to prove they have the strength. Isn't this pointless?! Admitting you need help or a favour is not weak, it is one of the strongest things you can possibly do. If we can just change our mindset to be more willing to accept help, we would all be so much more joyful. So, please, the next time you're thinking that you need help with something, ask for it. It will make you feel lighter. Then the next time that someone offers to help you, how about telling them, thank you that's kind, and letting them help? I will also be practising what I preach, I promise.

What if you're worried about how someone will react if you ask for help? The very start of a conversation can create an atmosphere instantly, and I've found that the best possible way to create a good atmosphere when you're asking for help is to tell them that you need their skills. Identifying what it is that that person can do brilliantly that you need and telling them about it will really lift them up and fill them with joy. Imagine how special you can make someone feel if you tell them you need them. I love being told that I am a help.

So, let's put this into practice. Let's imagine you need help. You can't get to collect the kids in time. Maybe you're worried that your dog will be alone for too long. Or perhaps you just need someone's brain to unpick a difficult problem that you're facing at the moment. We have all found ourselves in one of these situations, if not all. Ask someone that you trust for help. Asking for a favour in this way will NOT make you look weak, it will help you AND will make the person you ask feel wanted, useful and good, too. Again, it's one of those double whammies of joy that I keep speaking about. So when you've been able to start accepting help from others, start offering it out to others too. Spread your joy everywhere.

• Be generous with *your* time

When people think about the word 'generous', they immediately think of giving money. But that's not the only thing you can give – being generous of spirit or generous with your time is vitally important. I don't mean you should spend the whole day doing things for others; no, I am not preaching that here at all. All I am saying is that generosity is something we can all do, you don't have to spend any money and if **YOU** are generous, you will spread the joy. It goes back to something I talked about much earlier in this book.

LISTENING

Believe it or not, properly listening is generous. If you ask someone how they are and listen to what they say instead of just answering with a generic 'good', then you are being generous with your time.

Volunteering is another way of being generous, or just offering help to a friend or a family member can be a very special thing to do. I know some words can alarm people, and rather strangely the words 'generous' and 'volunteering' do make bells ring in some people's heads, but please tell those bells to quieten down. It doesn't have to be a grand gesture, either; the act of offering a friend a lift somewhere is generous. Giving clothes or objects to a charity shop is also generous. Giving someone your last sweet is kind and generous. Giving someone your time is so important.

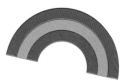

→ *Showbiz joy spreaders*

If I may, I would like to share with you two very starry stories
that have stayed with me for many years and still make me smile
hugely. Yes, they are showbizzy anecdotes, but in my job those
are the people I work with.

I have met an enormous number of incredibly famous people
and, yes, I still get excited when interviewing many of them.
When I think back over my years in TV and radio, I feel so lucky
about how many fabulous people I've met who simply want to
spread the joy. I was asked by a very dear friend recently who I
thought were the most fun famous joy-spreaders (after telling
him he said I should pop these two stories into this book), and
while I could list a massive line-up of the biggest showbiz
legends that I have met over the years, you don't want or need
a list of names here. So I have two fun tales to share with you,
which might sound like I am name-dropping (and I suppose I
am), but my friend DID ask me, so here goes. If you don't want
a couple of sweet showbiz tales, move on...

Billy Crystal and Tom Hanks are two of the kindest, funniest and
most uplifting people I've met. One of the biggest reasons behind
that is they are so generous with their time and they both want
to make people smile and feel joy. What a gift! I'll start with the
shortened version of meeting Tom Hanks. He was in the UK to
promote one of his movies (he's made so many that I can't
remember which one it was now!), and a press junket had been
set up – which is where all the TV and radio shows go along to a
hotel to chat to the stars and the team about the movie they're
promoting (just like that scene in *Notting Hill*). I had been
allocated ten minutes to go into the room to interview him,
which was tiny and packed with camera people, publicists and
make-up artists crowding around him. We started our chat and
laughed together as I asked the usual film-related questions.
Then I asked him to sing the rap that he'd sung in his 1988
movie *Big* (you may know the one and if not, you must watch
that film – it's a delight). He did sing it and I joined in (or tried
to). One of the people in charge was a very strict American

woman who, at this point, stood up, glared at me and told me to wind up my conversation; I'd had my ten minutes and I wasn't allowed even a minute more. But Tom stood up and said (very politely) that he thought she should let me stay. Everyone started whispering and then yessing to Tom, and I stayed. We laughed, sang and giggled together for thirty minutes. I am sure he'd done that many times before with many interviewers, but in asking me to stay, he made me feel special and so happy. He was polite, kind, warm, welcoming and funny. Those are the qualities that help spread joy. They are simple things that we are all capable of.

Now for the next name-drop moment and onto the other person that I mentioned, Billy Crystal. My encounter with Billy was quite a few years ago now. I met him on a breakfast show that I hosted where I had to recreate 'that' famous 'yes, yes, yes!' scene from *When Harry Met Sally* (you know the one: 'I'll have what she's having!'); he kept brilliantly in character and continued to play Harry perfectly with a straight face (I cannot tell you how embarrassed I felt because I was there with HIM doing THAT scene on British breakfast telly). Boy oh boy, I was a huge fan of his, and that was a surreal moment. I enjoyed our chat so much and, to my delight, after the interview, he said he wanted to stay longer and just hang around. He knew that I was enjoying his company, so he told his publicist that he wanted to stay. We chatted and chatted, and during that time he shared a story about his grandmother farting that to this day still makes me cry laughing. His impression of her was genius. He totally brought her to life and we laughingly both decided that we were related because we giggled crazily at the same things. Even once the show finished that morning he hung around, as I had cheekily asked him if we could possibly record a longer interview for a Christmas special. So he stayed and nattered some more, and I will never, ever forget that morning. Just a little aside – my all-time most favourite film is and was, even before meeting him, *When Harry Met Sally*. For me, this had been so huge and it still fills me with such joy to this day. I am absolutely sure he has no recollection of that morning, but I do!

By the way, you can watch Billy Crystal's brilliantly funny one-man show on Netflix where he talks so beautifully about his family and does touching impressions of them all, just like he did with me on that day. My family and I have watched it a few times and it's joyful and reminds me of the morning I spent with him. He has funny bones and he wants to make the person with him feel that you're in on the joke. He was so generous with his laughter.

Neither of these people had to spend extra time with me, but they chose to because they knew I was enjoying being with them. Generosity is such a huge way to spread joy. I know that many people will say that it's easy to be generous when you have money or are happy, but being generous isn't about money, it's about being generous with your spirit, your warmth and your laughs.

So be as generous with your time as you can be. Don't burn yourself out by doing it, but do give it to anyone you can who looks as though they might benefit from some more of it.

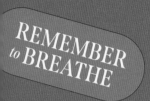
REMEMBER
to BREATHE

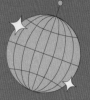

Conclusion

That's it! We've reached the end of this book but it's only the beginning of your journey towards sparking your own joyfulness and spreading this feeling around. You have taken part. You've walked, jumped, danced, sung, smiled, sniffed at some flowers, counted the leaves, said 'No' to some people and made more time for others. Hopefully, you have attempted the Tiny Tasks, and I am absolutely certain that, having done all of these things, you will be feeling so much lighter.

You may be wondering what comes next. This book is for dipping into again and again. Do you have a pencil? If not, please try to find one, and then draw in this book. Circle the parts that have helped you most and come back to them whenever you feel the need to. If there are some Tasks you didn't do when you were first reading the book, please do go back and try them now – I promise they will be helpful. Put bookmarks or Post-its on your favourite ones to remind yourself to do them, or, even better, stick these somewhere where you can't possibly avoid them to make sure that you

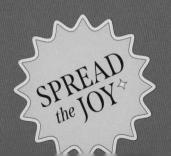
SPREAD
the JOY

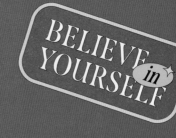

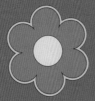

are making time for your Tiny Tasks every day. If you've finished them all and are remembering to slot them into your day regularly, why not push yourself a little further? Set yourself a new goal that's a bit more of a stretch for you in each area.

The final thing that I'd like to ask you to do after closing this book is to please do me and yourselves a huge favour and go out into the world smiling. Remember, you are not being judged, and there are no rules.

In this book I have held your hand from a distance and told you that you can do it – that you can prioritise yourself, the things that you like to do and re-awaken your inner child while STILL being an adult and feeling immense joy. Now, it's time for you to take what you've learnt forwards. You too can be bursting with fabulousness and joy and can help others to feel joy and fabulousness – it all starts when you look inside, appreciate the little things, break the rules, express yourself and spread the joy.

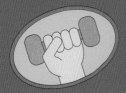

✳ Helpful resources

This is a list of charities and other resources that are there to provide support if you need it.

Cancer Research UK: Cancer Research UK provides information for anyone affected by any kind of cancer. Call the nurse helpline on 0808 800 4040. (www.cancerresearchuk.org)

Childhood Bereavement Network: The Childhood Bereavement Network is a specialist membership organisation, working together to support bereaved children and young people. (www.childhoodbereavementnetwork.org.uk)

Cruse: Cruse provides free care and bereavement counselling to people suffering from grief. Call the helpline on 0808 808 1677. (www.cruse.org.uk)

Mind: Mind provides free resources and information on various mental health conditions, and advice on how to get support. (www.mind.org.uk)

NHS website: You can find information and advice on health conditions, symptoms, healthy living, medicines and how to get help on the NHS website. (www.nhs.uk)

NHS 111: If you need to speak to a medical professional but can't get through to your GP, you can ring 111 for medical advice and reassurance over the phone.

The Samaritans: The Samaritans provides a free confidential helpline, 24 hours a day, if you need someone to talk to. Call 116 123. (www.samaritans.org)

WAY (Widowed and Young): WAY is a peer-to-peer support group for people who were aged 50 or under when their partner died. Call 0300 201 0051. (www.widowedandyoung.org.uk)

Acknowledgements

This may be the hardest part of the book to write because I like to say thank you. As you'll have read about in the book, it's something I think is very important. I have so many thank yous, but I will simply start by saying thank you to everyone for supporting me, for letting me follow my dreams and for laughing with and at me. My gorgeous team at HQ, including Lisa, who believed in me and this book from the very beginning. Louise and Alice, for bringing my imagination to life. Thank you to the fabulous, strong women who held my hand while getting the book out there: Sian, Rachael, Claire, Steph and Tamara and not forgetting Abi. Also, my blooming fantastic agent, George Ashton, who shares my love of life and is a joy-spreader. My husband, David, whom I love so deeply. Thank you for putting up with my craziness and for loving me like no one else has ever done. My two beautiful daughters, Libbi-Jack and Amelie, who let me sing musical theatre songs to them first thing in the morning and never tell me to be quiet. They both fill my heart with total joy. And a huge thank you to each and every one of my truly amazing, wonderful friends. I am blessed to have the dearest, kindest and most loyal friends, who have held my hand throughout my life. And lastly my mum and dad, who told me how important dreams are and to never give up on mine.

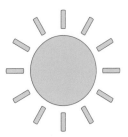

✴ About the author

Gaby Roslin is one of the country's favourite radio and TV presenters. She has hosted *The Big Breakfast*, *Children in Need*, *The Terry and Gaby Show* and many other shows for the BBC, Channel 4, ITV and Channel 5. She currently hosts shows including BBC Radio London, BBC One's Morning Live and is a regular presenter on BBC Radio 2. She has more than 200,000 followers on Instagram, where she regularly posts her Spread the Joy content, and has her own podcast *That Gaby Roslin Podcast: Reasons to be Joyful*.

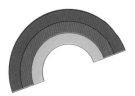

• Index